PRAISES FOR FORGETTING TO REMEMBER

Deb Kline has written an honest and heart-rending account of how childhood sexual abuse affected her life. From before the time of forgetting to beyond the time of remembering, her book is filled with the stark and harrowing details of what it means to be a survivor. That she can write such a book allows all of us to realize that it is possible to recover from horrible childhood trauma and, in the end, be able to truly heal. Ultimately, this is a story of hope.

Candida Maurer, PhD

If you ever wanted evidence that artistry can heal, look no further than Deb Kline's *Forgetting to Remember*. The story tells Kline's path from incest and rape—with all the brokenness and shattered sense of herself that this abuse wrought—towards the wholeness that years of increasing self-awareness and work with professionals in western and eastern medicine make possible. The narrative itself is riveting, but more arresting is the sheer beauty of the story's form, and of the sentences that, through sophisticated metaphors and stylistic shapes, catch readers up in lyricism.

Kline's artistry is everywhere. Whether by using poetry at the beginning of each chapter to forecast events and reflections to come or to acknowledge difficult truths understood after struggle, or whether by invoking the joyful memory of her 87-year-old Great Grandma playing kickball or the pleasure Deb took in learning how to tie her own shoes or ride a bike (not all her childhood events were harrowing), the author captures our hearts.

She also uses her phenomenal gift of creating absolutely apt metaphors to bring her struggles to life, casting the terrain of her life as volcanic fields with molten rock, or of tidal waves and powerful waterfalls, or of being at the wrong latitude and longitude on the planet such that she shouts to herself, "Correct your coordinates!"

Kline has turned her story into art, enfolding herself in art's healing powers, and taking readers along for the illuminating and transcendent ride.

Nancy Jones, PhD, Director Emeritus, Writing Resource Center, University of Iowa College of Law

There are life events that can wound and wound deeply. In *Forgetting to Remember*, Deb Kline speaks eloquently and courageously to her personal experience of sexual abuse in childhood and its ramifications for her life. Journeys of healing are filled with ambiguity and paradox. This is the case in Deb's story in which the wounding itself holds the source of healing.

The psyche is very adept in helping one to survive terrain which otherwise could be over-whelming and unbearable, especially to a developing child. This terrain can be locked deeply within the unconscious mind until circumstances arrive that begin to unlock it. In this book, Deb shares the journey of remembering and then "re-membering." This entails the long process of taking disturbing sensations, flashes of memory, images, and thoughts, working with them over many years, and coming to an exploration and understanding of her own backstory. This allows the emergent knowledge to guide her healing process.

Deb describes her own journey of healing—what happened, how she responded, and the ways help came, noting what helped and what didn't. She sought outer resources while developing inner ones such as learning when to let go and opening to her own intuitive wisdom of what was right for her. It is the latter which served her especially well. This is a story of healing, not cure. For can anyone of us ever be cured of our human condition or our particular frailties and penchants for seeking ourselves outside of ourselves? This is Deb's story of her movement toward personal wholeness and using all of what life had given her, bidden and unbidden, to become a woman unto herself, one who knows her unique place in the world and her connection to everything and everyone.

Forgetting to Remember, an engrossing and well-written book, will be valuable not only to those who have suffered childhood sexual abuse but also to anyone who wants to understand what true healing embodies.

Kathy Reardon, RN, MS, Spiritual Director,
Co-founder of the PrairieFire program

Deb Kline is a gifted woman who courageously shares her experience of childhood incest and teenage rape and the healing journey that followed. Her engaging story describes the ups and downs and twists and turns she weathered to reassemble a life interrupted and shattered by sexual abuse and assault. The author's account of being required to learn music theory and sight-read musical scores, rather than "play by heart what I felt in my soul," becomes a powerful metaphor for how healing ultimately comes from within.

For those beginning a similar journey, *Forgetting to Remember: A Healer's Journey of Surviving and Thriving* can serve as a beacon of hope. For mental health providers, Deb's story offers valuable insights into what is, and is not, helpful if they choose to walk alongside those on a similar journey.

J. Jeffrey Means, MDiv, PhD,
Author of Trauma & Evil: Healing the Wounded Soul

As a licensed, HSP psychologist for 35 years, I have seen over a thousand clients and done over 10,000 psychological evaluations during my career. I always tried to be faithful to my clients and frequently had to deal with the scourge of sexual abuse and misogyny in our country and culture. Deb Kline tells her story of an innocent child betrayed by her family. She writes about the repressed and rediscovered traumas of her childhood and youth, portraying how in trauma part of our mind can shut down and not allow us to acknowledge the horrors and monsters that we face. She does so with clarity, conviction, and amazing empathy to the perpetrators and enablers of her remembered abuse. After a long journey, Deb has swum over to the other side. Hers is a story of great pain and eventual healing through much work and suffering. This is a tale that shows the indomitable resiliency of the human spirit.

Arthur H. Konar, PhD, Licensed Psychologist

Deb Kline, author of the moving memoir *Forgetting to Remember*, does not shield us from the truth. In the opening pages, she details the incest her father perpetrated, and in the next chapter, she describes her experience of stranger rape. Neither does she abandon us as we attempt to make sense of this abuse. In a keen, perceptive voice, honed by years of reflection, Deb anticipates what we will want to know: How did she move from the traumatized child to the aware and inspirational adult she is today?

We learn how she buries, then relives, this trauma as current day events trigger her. That begins her amazing journey, fitting together the pieces of her life she describes as a jigsaw puzzle with missing, ill-fitting parts.

Whether other survivors adopt her specific strategies is less the point. Readers well see Deb's determination and drive to be whole as she finally declares herself the CEO of her own re-creation.

You may not have experienced sexual abuse or other childhood trauma, but in telling her story, Deb lets us walk along alongside her and in doing so gives us wisdom to accompany those on similar journeys.

Diane Glass, author of The Heart Hungers for Wildness

Victims/survivors will feel fully understood, and therapists and others will gain new understandings throughs Deb's clear descriptions of incest and stranger rape, of forgetting, and then recovering memories. Deb employs playful as well as powerful prose to illuminate how forgetting works and recovery can happen: finding the right treatment team, accepting spousal support, processing anger effectively, forgiving with boundaries, and arriving at spiritual integration. She emphasizes that each recovery journey is individual, but the universals she shares will normalize the need for healing and comfort those with the same lived experience. I will be loaning copies to clients, knowing Deb's story can benefit them, even if they skip over the two sexual violence descriptions. Therapists will appreciate her sophistication, while all readers will enjoy her friendly voice, stories of good relationships, musical creativity, and joy.

Suzanne Zilber, PhD,
Psychologist specializing in trauma treatment for 30 years

FORGETTING TO REMEMBER

Forgetting to Remember

A Healer's Journey of Surviving and Thriving

Deb Kline

Zion Publishing

Copyright © 2020 Deb Kline

All rights reserved. No part of this publication may be reproduced, stored in a retrieval system, or transmitted in any form or by any means—electronic, mechanical, photocopy, recording, or any other—except for brief quotations in printed reviews, without the prior permission of the publisher.

Cover photograph by Kendal Kline
Cover drawing by Deb Kline
Interior drawing by Deb Kline
Poetry by Deb Kline
Photograph on p. 345 by Kendal Kline

ISBN: 978-1-7368640-3-6

Library of Congress Control Number: 2020924827

Published by
Zion Publishing
Des Moines, Iowa

Important

Trigger Warning: This book contains explicit scenes of sexual abuse encounters. Please read at your discretion, prioritizing your own self-care. If at any time you feel overwhelmed by your own trauma, please: call the free and confidential National Sexual Assault Hotline, available 24 hours all days, at **1-800-656-4673**; or visit **www.rainn.org** for chat options.

Disclaimer 1: For the purpose of anonymity, the names, identifying characteristics, occupations, or places of residence of family members, childhood friends, teachers, and care providers may have been changed, and gender-neutral pronouns (they/them/their) used. The memories of events herein may or may not reconcile with those of family, friends, teachers, and care providers, but are factual accounts true to the author's recollections.

Disclaimer 2: This book depicts one woman's healing journey. It is not intended to be used as a how-to manual for individual healing or to replace advice from medical experts or professional counselors.

Hear Deb's Music

References are made in the text to original copyrighted music albums and songs by the author. Listen or download for free at **www.debkline.com**. If you download any materials, the author requests that you make in-kind donations to human service non-profit organizations of your choosing, as your circumstances allow. All rights reserved. Do not use without the artist's permission.

See Deb's Artwork

References are made in the text to original SoulCollage® artwork by the author. These images are available for viewing purposes only, to illustrate the SoulCollage® process. SoulCollage® cards are not to be sold, traded, or bartered. Do not reproduce, copy, share, or save these images. You can find these images at **www.debkline.com** (password = forgetting).

Contents

I remember black	
Prologue	7
Do you know what a little girl said to me?	
Introduction	11

Section I

The Remembered and Forgotten Childhood

Raggedy Ann	
1. A Not So Uncommon Occurrence	21
She waits under stone	
2. Denial is Stronger than Memory	47
And the faster the world spins...	
3. Joyride	59
A cold, dark room	
4. The Shadow Monster	87

Section II

My Normal Family with Abnormal Me

Mirror, mirror on the wall	
5. What is Wrong with Me?	95
Stuck on a music box	
6. The Heart of a Musician	103
I Lurk as the Loch Ness Monster	
7. Coming of Age	121
Here she comes now	
8. Cinnamon & Dawn	133

But there were birthday cakes
9. ON A GIVEN SUNDAY   **141**

Hazel's Lamp
10. MY TWIN SOUL   **151**

As time went on we stumbled
11. A RUDDERLESS YOUNG ADULTHOOD   **167**

Section III

Exposed to the Light

There's something new
12. HAPPILY EVER AFTER   **207**

Once she forgot to remember
13. FORGETTING TO REMEMBER   **235**

My porcupine tongue
14. ANGER: MY SUPERPOWER   **249**

I will sow seeds of self-nurturing
15. GROUNDING AND UNGROUNDING   **265**

I am sitting
16. THE WOUNDED HEALER   **295**

I have faith in an embracing universe
17. A TIME TO THRIVE   **311**

Every little piece of me is in every little piece of you
AFTERWARD:
HEALING POTENTIAL ABOUNDS   **329**

Memorial Shells
ACKNOWLEDGMENTS:
WITH THANKS, PRAISE, AND GRATITUDE   **339**

This book is dedicated to sexual abuse victims and survivors.

May you find a touchstone here to lead you back to yourself and embrace yourself fully.

May you thrive.

I remember black,
You remember blue.
I am the crack in the family photograph.
I am the scratch in the record skipping,
  Skipping,
    Back to the beginning again.

I was one child,
But I remember two.
One was the blonde pixie pictured here.
The other girl went screaming,
  Screaming,
    To where only dogs can hear her.

You rose with the sun,
I woke with the moon.
You danced with your shadow,
That was me.
You couldn't see the stars tripping,
  Tripping,
    For all your bright beauty.

You reflected light,
I absorbed the dark.
You barely glimpsed me on cloudy days.
I was the one in the corner waving,
  Waving,
    "Hey, wait for me!"

Prologue

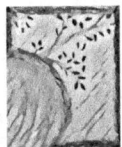

Why are children afraid of the dark? Is fear of night and shadows handed down to us from adult to child through the generations? Is it a universal theme to have monsters lurking at bedtime, hiding underneath the bed, waiting behind the closet door, peering from outside the window?

The children's television program, *Sesame Street*, addresses children's fear of monsters by creating beloved puppet characters (Oscar the Grouch, Cookie Monster, Grover, Count von Count, and more recently Elmo, Zoe, and Rosita), bringing them into the daylight and casting them as friends.

As a child, even after watching my puppet monster friends on TV, reading their tales in books, and playing with them as stuffed animals, I was still afraid of the other monsters after dark, the scary ones I imagined lingering in the shadows at night in my bedroom waiting to devour me. Adults reassure children that monsters aren't real, that they are imaginary and live only in our heads.

But what about the real monster in the dark, the father in my bed, his body beneath my covers, his breath on my neck, his hands inside my nightgown? First, I was sworn to secrecy, then I was gaslighted (manipulated to question my own perceptions), led to forget. I second-guessed myself. No one wants to believe such monstrous happenings, least of all me. I must be mistaken. It must have been a bad dream, a nightmare. Things like that don't happen in quaint neighborhoods, in nice homes, in Christian households, in good families—not under our roof. How could that be possible? It was deniable from the outside looking in, and from the inside looking out if you believed adults over children. Everyone did back then. "Respect your elders." "Do what I say, not what I do." "Be a good girl and do as you're told."

It will become clearer throughout my story just how the incest narrative vanished and reappeared, how it was both known and unknown to the individuals involved, and how denying the real monster outside of me created a real monster within me, a Shadow Monster.

*Do you know what a little girl said to me?
I tried to tell you, like I tried to tell them too,
But no one would listen…
     guess it don't matter anyway.*

*Why get mad at me? I didn't do this thing.
This unthinkable thing was done to me.
I couldn't stop it, and I often wished I'd die,
But no one could listen…
     guess it don't matter anyway.*

*There was a Monster who lived in our house.
He was the Beast and I his Beauty,
But he plucked my beauty out from
     right between my legs,
And no would hear him,
No one could hear him,
No one heard him…
     but me.*

Introduction

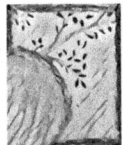

Incest. I wish it were uncommon, but it's not. A trusted relative stealthily inserts it into a child's routines, like changing into play clothes, putting on a swimsuit, drying off after bathing, cuddling in while reading, snuggling up while sleeping, adding fondling when something else is also happening and when no one else is around, making it as common for a child as daily life.

Incest. The act is abhorrent, taboo, so families blur their vision with excuses, hide their truths with denial, condemn both perpetrator and victim to silence, and it remains invisible, unseen, unacknowledged, unheard. It scares me to think how many children in how many homes are not safe, yet nobody knows. I was not safe in my own home. Nobody knew.

Incest. According to The National Sexual Violence Resource Center,[1] one in four girls and one in six boys, are sexually abused before turning eighteen years of age. I am one of those girls. Our sexual perpetrators are 96 percent male. One third of the victims, like me, are abused by a family member. Still, "Only 12 percent of child sexual abuse is ever reported to the au-

---

1   www.nsvrc.org/statistics

thorities."[2] I am in the 88 percent, as my father-daughter incest has never been reported.

The father-daughter incest I endured was our family secret. The secret was so furtive, in fact, that I blocked it out of my memory for nearly three decades, limping through life as if I were not wounded, steering my life as if there were no roadblocks, unaware that my life was anything but normal. I started recovering the incest memories at age 29, and finally remembered all of the childhood sexual abuse encounters by age 33.

It's a stretch to call my father's incest a family secret. Without identifying them by name, my immediate family numbered five: Mom, Dad, Bigbro—not quite three years older than me, Me, and Lilbro—just past three years younger than me. I'm sure neither of my brothers ever knew about the incest. I have no memories of them in or around my dad's "Special Game," as he called it. The abuse happened behind closed doors, sometimes in the bathroom, more often in the privacy of my childhood bedroom, either at night when my brothers would have been sleeping, or by day when they weren't around. My dad only initiated his game when I was upstairs, when we were alone, and when he could hear potential intruders, thus being assured that his believable fibs would lie unquestioned. Bigbro and Lilbro, like the rest of the outside world, had no reason to suspect a thing. Our public persona was that of a happy, ordinary, middle class, Christian family.

The paradox of my dad engaging in father-daughter incest with me was that the man who was supposed to love his daughter more than any other girl in the

---

2   www.nsvrc.org/statistics

world, and who was supposed to protect her at all costs, violated that oath by violating me. The paradox includes many unanswerable questions. Where was his unconditional love for me, his child? What made him act in ways he knew were unforgivable? Can I in any way reconcile his contradictory behavior? Do I and can I love someone who defiled me?

Looking back to my early childhood, I always remembered being Daddy's Little Girl, with all the fun-loving innocence that expression portrays. Post age 33, I have a new timeline of memories.

My memory lines are like an AM/FM radio. The Always Memories (AM) are on the old timeline and have always been accessible to me, and they include all the events of my life, post-birth to now, minus the sexual abuse episodes. Like the AM radio, it existed first, so it's always been around, but its frequencies don't carry complex sounds well.

The Forgotten Memories (FM) are on a new timeline, and they exclusively hold all the sexual abuse memories that were only accessible after being uncovered in adulthood. Like the FM radio, it existed second, so it is more recent, and its frequency can carry more complex sounds further, with more clarity.

When I recall events, I must intentionally switch from one timeline to the other, because my Always Memories and my Forgotten Memories exist separately. I must choose which timeline to tune into to retrieve a memory. The radio must be set to either AM or FM to designate the station one wants to hear, but one cannot listen to both AM and FM at the same time, because they use different frequencies. So it is with my memories, since I recovered them between the ages of 29 and 33, and they remain separate today.

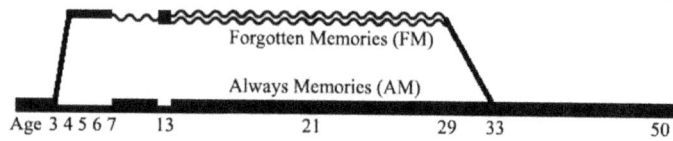

In this book, when I share memories that have always been with me, I will indicate AM for the Always Memory setting. If I want to share memories previously forgotten, remembered by me only later when I was an adult, I will indicate FM for the Forgotten Memories setting. In my mind, the two lines are parallel, as if I've led two lives. I cannot combine the two timelines into one. Instead, the lines reside one above the other. The new timeline, appearing out of thin air, hovers, floating over the old, and I can clearly see the obvious points where they would overlap, but I can't get them to intersect. It is only from age 33 forward that the AM and FM lines remerge into a single timeline again. From that point on, I have a single life, but looking back prior to age 29, my life looks like this double image diagram, the wavy lines representing the splintered parts of me hidden within—hidden by the Shadow Monster.

I am writing now in my 50s, a half-century after the incest began, for now I can speak my history with power, now I can contribute my voice to expose the hidden epidemic of childhood sexual abuse, now I can say the words incest and rape without self-shame, now I can embody my healed soul.

I write to share my story alongside stories untold. I speak this truth among truths still silenced in order to give kinship to the kindred who are feeling alone, to offer hope of healing where healing seems impossible. Healing is a private journey, a journey that needs its own time and space, its own boundaries to ensure safety, its own privacy that may be too precious to share. If you, too, Dear Reader, have endured sexual abuse, whatever your journey looks like, wherever you are on your journey, however isolated you may feel, you are not alone.

Section I

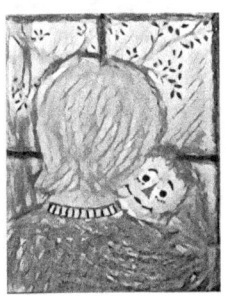

The Remembered and Forgotten Childhood

Raggedy Ann

*She sits in her rocker, (rocking her Annie):
a girl of six in a pixie.
Thunder shudders her spine erect
as she blinks back icy fingers
streaking down the bedroom window.*

Annie can't sleep...
Lightening blinded her awake.

But the pixie girl hugs Annie
with ribs and words:

"Tree arms don't beckon ghosts,
but dance to heaven's drums;
the holler you hear is not of death—
a silly angel stubbed her wing;
I don't know why
God takes pictures
during thunderstorms."

CHAPTER I

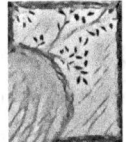

A NOT SO UNCOMMON OCCURRENCE

AM (Always Memory): Shady Lane is a quiet, north-south street, only two blocks long, that runs the length of a hillcrest. The east-west streets on either side slope down and away, as does the middle street dividing the neighborhood into two halves. Mature oak and maple trees run the length of its sidewalks on either side. My house nestles on the west side of the street near the north end. Narrow and tall—2 ½ stories with a peaked attic—and painted white with green trim, it has a full length, screened-in porch running along its front. A wooden bench swing, a spot I prize, is suspended at one end, hanging by chain links. Sometimes I swing alone, holding my Raggedy Ann doll while imagining us on adventures far, far away from home; sometimes with my brothers, pretending we're on a plane swinging high and fast in the clouds to a distant land; sometimes with girlfriends, giggling about how to avoid catching cooties from boys; and sometimes with Great-Grandma, tucked safely under her arm, barely swinging, cherishing each other's presence without words.

The house has a full basement, unfinished, that circles an ominous, flaming furnace my brothers and I pretend is a monster. To one side, Dad's tool bench and ham radio equipment take up half the dank room (dubbed the dungeon), where he spends hours hiding out, tinkering with broken gadgets or clicking Morse code to people all across the globe. The opposite area from the dungeon serves as laundry, stashed with the wringer washer and rinse tubs my Mom fills and drains every Monday. Clotheslines, secured to the rafters, sag under the weight of drying sheets and clothes on rainy or winter days.

The neighboring houses are similar, though not identical—newly built in 1918, over four and a half decades old, and getting older while my family resides here. Surrounded by grass-covered yards, front to back, with flowers bordering the perimeters, the homes shelter traditional, white, middle-class families, with two or more children per house, spilling out the doors onto the lawns—children that become a crew of playmates for my brothers and me.

Here I am, a brown-eyed blonde with hair cropped short in a pixie and contrasting brunette eyebrows. Average height for my age, I have a slender build and am active and agile as I chase to keep up with my older brother and his buddies. Even though my favorite toy is my Raggedy Ann, and I have a variety of other dolls, I choose to play with trucks and Legos just as often. I pride myself on being a tomboy, climbing trees, playing in the dirt, and wrestling with my dad and brothers.

Our front door catches the morning sun. As I enter past the porch swing, on through to the entryway, a wooden stairway rises along the right wall to the second floor. A railing leads to the top and wraps around at two right angles to line a small open portion of the upstairs hallway. We kids enjoy this perch, peeking down through the spindles to spy on the first-floor dwellers below.

I remember that twice Lilbro jutted his head through one of the gapped openings to get a better look down and trapped his head. He couldn't pull it back out for his ears, though he tried. With the first incident, my amused dad repressed his laughs as he fetched his toolbox, removed one of the spindles to free him, and then fixed the spindle back into its proper place. When the incident repeated, my annoyed dad insisted that this was the last time he would pry him free, warning Lilbro that—if he got his head stuck again—he would have to stay trapped forever. Dad's threat worked, likely because Lilbro believed it sincere. Being unable to tell whether he was joking or not was a common confusion for us with Dad.

At the top of the staircase, a dim, narrow hallway is lined with five doors—to a linen closet, three bedrooms and a bathroom. Most of my childhood, my brothers bunk together, and I have my own bedroom. I enjoy peeking out the east-facing window with its sky view over the neighborhood. When it's hard to sleep because the summer light lingers past bedtime, I can both observe the scurrying bodies of the older kids and hear them shouting pronouncements of, "Olly olly oxen free," as they play Kick the Can in the street below. I giggle as I imagine a stampede of oxen, each with the name of Olly, galloping freely down Shady

Lane, their thundering hooves turning west down the center hill and running far, far away.

Back on the main floor entryway, a supporting wall divides two sets of open rooms. Straight ahead, the kitchen area opens onto an eat-in dining nook with a table and chairs—six seats, one for each of us with one to spare. The spare chair is often occupied by my Raggedy Ann doll, who gets her own tableware setting. Here is where we eat all our family meals—breakfast, lunch, and supper.

Mom isn't hungry in the morning, so breakfast is a free-for-all of whatever cereal boxes Dad puts on the table. A coveted, freshly unsealed box signals a new toy prize, so we mad-grab for the package to thrust our hands into the sugarcoated morsels—victory bestowed to the first fist to clutch the cellophane-wrapped surprise. With Dad off to work, Mom fixes us lunch, my favorite being Kraft Macaroni and Cheese or peanut butter and jelly sandwiches. When Dad returns home from work, the hot meal Mom prepares is ready at five o'clock. We wash our hands, settle into our places, say our grace ("God is great, God is good, let us thank him for our food, Amen") and dig in, eating our fill, but saving room for dessert.

To the left of the entry on the main floor, a wide-open space leads to the living room. The black-and-white TV with rabbit ears sits in one corner, and a console record player and AM/FM radio rest along an opposite wall. A long brown couch and some modern-style armchairs line the perimeter walls, with dining chairs scrunched in for holiday dinners and birthday celebrations to hold both sides of our local extended family of grandmas and great-grandmas, along with generations of aunts and uncles, and before long a bunch of cousins. The only grandpa is my dad's dad, but he unofficially adopts my mom's siblings as his own children and my cousins on my mom's side as his vicarious grandkids. Everyone calls him Grandpa, and the two sides of my parents' families are so entwined that, for the longest time, I don't realize who is and is not blood-related, not that it matters. We're all family.

The living room opens to the official dining room beyond, where Mom's upright piano sits against the interior wall and, in the opposite corner by a south window, resides Petey, Mom's green parakeet, in a wire cage with a perch and a trapeze swing. His cheerful chirping brightens the room. My brothers and I try to teach him to talk, "Polly, want a cracker?" but he doesn't ever say a word. We also get to take turns refilling his food and water dishes, but Mom is always the one to refresh the newspapers on the bottom of the birdcage—she doesn't want Petey to escape.

I sometimes sit by myself beside the cage, talking to the trapped Petey, alone in his cage, only able to flit, not fly as he sees other birds outside the window freely soaring in the sky, living their best bird lives with no trappings, singing songs of freedom he can only dream of. What if just once I let him out? I could claim I made a mistake and apologize. It's worth the risk of a spanking or getting grounded to my bedroom for Petey to fly free, however briefly.

One day, when the coast is clear, I commit the forbidden oopsies and prop open the cage door. Petey hops to the opening, pokes his head through looking this way and that, then bursts free—fluttering feathers and cheerful chirps—Petey flies, liberated and soaring, albeit indoors. Flapping wings dive through the dining room and swoop through the den, buzzing Bigbro's head. He ducks as Petey veers past him in a stunt turn toward the living room. "Petey's out! Petey's out!" Bigbro shouts, spoiling my fun.

Dad, frazzled and frantic, bursts from his dungeon, launching into a free-for-all chase in pursuit of the flapping bird. He leaps, the parakeet tweets flitting along the ceiling, and I witness the battle of wills between escapee and captor. I'm rooting for Petey. Dad exacerbates the commotion, reacting to the drama as a life and death emergency, nothing else mattering in the moment as he focuses solely on snatching the bird and forcing it back into captivity. "Gotcha!" Dad exclaims as he wins, clutching Petey in his grasp. "Back you go into the cage where you belong. Game over!" he says. I sigh, sad and heavy, as I watch Petey imprisoned again, his independence thwarted, his rebellion halted, and life goes back to normal.

Then one day, I notice Petey lying in the bottom of his cage. I get Mom to show her, "Mom, Petey's sleeping. Wake up, Petey! It's time for breakfast."

"He's not going to wake up, Honey. He went to heaven," Mom said, and I watched her slip his limp body in a shoebox that she buried in the backyard.

I didn't cry for poor Petey. But I was sad that he never got to be a real bird, never felt the wind in his feathers, never tasted fresh worms for a meal, never gathered twigs to make a nest, never found a mate. He just existed alone in his cage, and for what? He was a pretty possession whose purpose was to amuse his captors by singing for his supper, and all the while, he was expected to be content behind bars—the only escape being death and burial in a box. But at least now, his spirit is free, soaring around in birdie heaven. I promise myself, when I grow up, I will never have a pet bird.

The opposite end of the formal dining room opens to the den. A wooden toy box with a hinged lid sits by a couch with all of our childhood treasures (blocks, Barbies, GI Joes, Legos, trucks, Hot Wheels race tracks and cars, Lincoln Logs) just waiting for my brothers and me to play with them. A bookshelf holds everything that won't fit into the toy box: my favorite board games (Candy Land and Chutes and Ladders), puzzles, coloring books and crayons, and a slew of children's books. The den holds a kid's paradise.

Inevitably, the toys and games spill out of the den and onto the dining room floor. Mom tolerates the mess as long as we are actively playing, but as soon as we are done, everything must be returned to its proper place, back into the toy box or onto the shelves. Picking up afterward is never as much fun as playing, and it seems to take forever, but it's what we do to keep this room tidy because it also holds Dad's office. Dad's desk and bookcase are squished to one side of the playroom after Lilbro is born. My bedroom takes over where his office used to be. This rearrangement is designed for my brothers and me to have separate bedrooms. When Dad's desk and bookcase are moved downstairs, the den serves as both an office and a playroom.

From the den, one can either circle around through where it is connected to the eat-in kitchen area or go out the back door into the back yard. The backyard has a white picket fence wrapping around the perimeter, dividing it from the neighbors' yards. A giant oak tree reaches its branches wide and high into the sky. Its trunk is broad enough that my arms can't encircle it, even when I join hands with Bigbro around the base of the tree.

One summer, my dad builds a tower fort in the backyard for us kids to play on. Four tall pillars support a high platform with railings. A ladder runs straight up along one side to climb. Underneath the platform, he hangs a single, slat-seat swing. It is mostly a father-son project for Bigbro and Dad to do together, but I still get to help and am able to hammer some nails into the boards all by myself, even if Dad straightens out a few when I am done. Lilbro is just a baby and too little to help. When the tower is finished, I enjoy times spent swinging and singing in the backyard underneath the elevated platform and climbing up to enjoy the bird's nest view while spying on neighboring yards.

FM (Forgotten Memory): In my 30s, I recall, during that same time, being Daddy's Little Girl in an eerie, sickening way. My dad knew what he was doing was wrong, because he kept it hidden and asked me to keep it secret, too. I was three when it began. He called what we are doing, "playing a Special Game." He invented it, and only he and I could play it.

It doesn't make sense to my three-year-old self why it has to be just the two of us. But Dad says so, so I go along. It's mostly just an undressing game, with me touching his boy part. His boy part is just like the ones my brothers have, only it is bigger, and it sticks straight out, rather than dangling down between his legs. Dad says his pointing boy part is a magic trick.

At first, I feel flattered by the singled-out attention. The Special Game indeed makes me feel special. It is fun to keep a secret that no one else in the whole wide world knows about except me and Dad—a special bond just between the two of us.

AM: I love bath time. In the brief window, when my brothers and I are still small, we can all three fit in the tub together. There are copious amounts of Mr. Bubble, enough to hide our plastic floating toys and to form into foamy beards and hats.

I search through the bubbles for my favorite toy, the Three Men in a Tub boat. It looks like a pint-sized, half whiskey barrel, with three weeble-wobble-shaped figurines, so each sibling can have one, with no need to share. It is from the nursery rhyme, "Rub a dub dub, three men in a tub…," but we say, "Rub a dub dub, three kids in a tub…," and giggle. After playing and getting clean, when the bubbles have dissipated, and the water turned cool, we pruney-skinned siblings are ready to get out. The three of us, freshly clean, take turns getting dried off. I have goosebumps and shiver, stepping onto the bathmat. Mom or Dad holds up the towel, wide open, and I run into the fuzzy cloth as it envelopes me, surrounding me in softness and hugs. Hands rub me dry from all sides at once, it seems, and I feel showers of affection before being ordered to put on my jammies and get ready for bed.

FM: One time, after my bath, I feel uncomfortable. Just Dad and I are in the bathroom. He reaches up through my legs from behind with the towel and lingers there. I wait. Finally, I have to tell him, I am dry down there now. He sheepishly shrugs and says, "Oh, okay," and finishes drying off the rest of me. He repeats this technique often enough to make me not want to let my dad dry me off anymore. I have another similar memory, where Dad is waiting with an open towel after my bath. I don't want to let him dry me off. As he stands in front of me waiting, I shout out down the hallway, "Mom, I want you to dry me off, please!"

She calls back, "I'm busy with your brothers! Let your dad do it! Where is he?"

"I'm right here," my dad calls back for her to hear. He looks hurt. We both know why I am hesitating.

"I'm big enough to dry myself now," I insist.

"Fine," he says, tosses me the towel, and leaves the bathroom.

I struggle to wrap the towel around me and pat myself dry before it falls to the floor. Rewrapping, shimmying and patting, I awkwardly towel-dry myself, having never done this before. I could have used help, but make do on my own.

AM: My best friend Erin (from the church nursery) and I are both three years old. One Sunday morning, amidst our usual snacking—napkins heaping with oyster crackers and dinky Dixie cups of orange Kool-Aid—Erin tells me she is going to start taking ballet lessons. My ears perk up, and my whole body tingles. Her mom has already purchased for her a pink leotard with matching tights and dance slippers. I am instantly envious and dying to take ballet lessons too. Never before have I wanted anything so much. Did I mention I'm only three? I bombard her with questions. Where will she take the lessons? A real dance studio. When do they start? In a few weeks. How often will she go? Once a week. I am determined to be a ballet dancer, too, just like Erin. But what if my parents don't let me? What if they say no?

I pick a time when my mom is alone, and, despite my angst, I summon the courage to ask her if I can take ballet lessons like Erin.

"It's now or never. Just do it," I think to myself, and then blurt out loud, in a rush of breath, "Mom, can I please, please, please, take ballet lessons? Erin's mom is letting her take them, and I want to take dancing lessons so bad!" My request hangs midair, as I await her response. My heart pounds in my tiny chest.

"Erin's taking ballet lessons? How do you know that?" Mom asks.

"Because Erin told me so. She already has a leotard, tights, and ballet slippers and everything." I'm nervous because the fate of my dancing career, which may never begin, is in her hands. One word, and it is all over. I don't want her to say no. Please, please, please don't say no!

"I'll think about it. Let me talk to Erin's mom. We'll have to see how much it costs."

I quickly bargain, "If you let me take dance lessons, I don't need to get any more birthday presents or Christmas presents ever again." That should save some money, I think. I'm still nervous while holding out for her final answer, but at least she didn't say no, not yet, and maybe, just maybe, she'll say yes.

The "yes" I'm so anxious to hear finally comes. "You won't be in the same dance school as Erin," Mom warns. Apparently, Erin's studio is too expensive.

"I don't care! I don't care! Just as long as I can take dance lessons! Yes! I'm going to be a dancer! I'm a dancer!" This is the best news of my young life, and I begin dancing on the spot, twirling like a ballerina all around the living room.

Now that I am officially going to be a ballerina, I have a new worry. Surely ballet dancers know how to tie their own ballet slippers. I don't even know how to tie my street shoes! I will be woefully embarrassed and look like a baby if I'm the only ballerina who can't tie her ballet slippers on the first day of class. I am desperate to learn to tie laces and don't have much time. Ballet class is about to begin (exactly when is unclear), but I know it will be soon. My mom brushes off my concern as me being silly and tells me that shoe tying isn't a necessary skill for dance class, so I beg my dad to teach me.

Dad tells Mom that I'm grown up enough to learn big-girl skills, and after a few tutorials, Dad sits in the living room chair and reads the newspaper, all the while letting me sit on the floor and practice tying and untying his shoes. His initial demonstration demystifies the magic trick.

"Crisscross the laces, then loop one under and pull them wide." His shoes are big, shiny, and brown with long thin laces, also brown. "Make sure there is no gap by pulling each lace tight. Now you're ready to tell a story. Here's the tree..." (he makes a loose loop with one of the laces and stands it up at the base of the crisscross), "and here's the rabbit" (he holds the remaining lace out straight). "The rabbit runs around the tree" (he winds the remaining lace around the base of the loop called the tree), "...and through the rabbit hole...," (he tucks the same lace through its own wind around the tree), "...and you pull the rabbit out by the ears." (He grasps the new loop formed by coming out of the hole and pulls both loops tight. What began as a tree is now the second rabbit ear.) "Abracadabra!"

I repeat the bunny story and actions, over and over again, until at last, it's my turn to exclaim, "Abracadabra!" I can do it! What a relief!

"That's my big girl!" Dad peeks around his newspaper and gives me a wink, and I, grinning and blushing, bask in his approval.

It's a bit trickier to tie my ballet slippers. The elastic laces are thin, stretchy, and short. I repeat the saying with the tree and the bunny until I can tie my ballet shoes, too.

On the first day of class, my stomach is aflutter with excitement beneath my purple leotard. Walking from the parking lot, I look up to see the giant sign with big letters. One day, I will be able to read it for myself ("Charlene's Dance Studio"), but not today. Beneath the sign is a glass double door. We enter the studio and are directed to a narrow side room just to the left. The coat room has long wooden benches running the length of each side, with cubbies built in underneath to store our street shoes. There are hooks for coats on the wall above each cubby, but they are empty. Coat season hasn't started yet. The room is abuzz with pint-sized pupils and full-sized parents.

"Rule number one of dance," I hear the teenager I will come to know as Lacy, the assistant, say, "you never, ever, ever, wear your street shoes into the dance studio. Only ballet slippers are allowed on the dance floor." She repeats this loudly, several times, as students and parents mill around her to get their names checked off her clipboard.

As I look around, all of the other parents are helping their first-time ballerinas put on their slippers, some even by placing their feet into the pink shoes for them. Not a single girl ties them herself, and none of them seem to care about being dependent on their parents for help.

I am taken aback by how helpless my peers appear to me. Am I really as young as they are? I guess Mom was right. I was worried about nothing. Instead of my shoe-tying skills being a matter of pride, in this setting, I feel conspicuously mature. My fear of being the only one who couldn't master shoe tying is not realized. Instead, I am glaringly alone in my newly acquired skill set. I shrug off a few compliments of amazement from both the kids and parents around me. It is a different kind of embarrassment, me not wanting to stand out as a shoe-tying show-off.

FM: At night, I have no choice whether or not I play the Special Game with Dad. He wanders into my room unannounced, whenever he likes, and snuggles into my bed alongside me. It's not every night, but his visits come in bunches, and then lapses, and then bunches again. The details of the fondling exchanges also blur together. I find it a blessing, when the memories return, that I have few detailed encounters to ponder.

The nighttime versions of the Special Game get interrupted and end abruptly, whenever we hear my mom get up and walk down the hallway to use the bathroom. As soon as the bathroom door closes, my dad sneaks back into his own bed before Mom is finished. I hear their muffled voices when she returns, my dad saying that I had a nightmare, or needed a drink of water, or some other lie, as to why he was in my room.

Both day and night, the Special Game commences enough times that I begin to attempt to prevent it from happening. Sometimes, if I pretend to be sleeping heavily and do not respond to Dad in my bed, he soon leaves. I can then breathe a sigh of relief and fall deeply asleep for real, for he never bothers me more than once a night. When he is gone, I know he won't be back again, at least not that evening.

For a brief time, I avoid getting up at night to use the bathroom because Dad will be waiting for me in my bed when I return. I must be waking him up, even though I tiptoe the length of the lighted hallway and carefully keep my bedroom door and the bathroom door from creaking. I stop drinking my bedtime glass of water. Despite refraining from liquid before bedtime, I still need to pee in the wee hours. I consider wetting the bed, but I am too old for that, so instead, I stand next to my bed and let the warm stream fill my panties and run down my leg into a puddle on the floor. It feels weird, but I wipe myself and the pee clean with the top of my underwear that is still dry. I toss the soiled panties on the corner floor of the closet and hop back into bed, wearing just my nightgown, bare underneath. My plan is working. Dad doesn't wake up.

My favorite custom, whenever Great-Grandma is at our house for an evening visit, is to have her tuck me and Raggedy Ann into bed. One night, I have not even had the chance to pick out my bedtime story yet when Great-Grandma wonders aloud, "What's that smell?" sniffing the air. Her nose detects my stash. I hope she won't open my closet door, but she does.

"What is this?" she gasps. Summoning my mom into my bedroom, she points to the soiled pile of underwear on the closet floor that she's sniffed out. I flush with embarrassment.

I can't explain the evidence honestly, so I quickly spin a lie, "I didn't want to wet the bed, so I got out, but I had to pee so bad I couldn't make it to the bathroom. I didn't want to tell anyone because I'm too old to wet my pants."

From then on, I am shamed into abandoning my bathroom-avoidance tactic. Whatever conversation kerfuffle follows, I am supposed to tell Mom right away when I wet myself so she can wash out my panties right away. I wonder if she is ever curious as to why this never happens again, why my excuse of urgently needing to pee suddenly disappears, and there are no soiled panties to wash. I return to trying to be as quiet as possible at night, tiptoeing my way to the bathroom. I add not clicking on the bathroom light and not flushing the toilet to my noiseless ritual. It sometimes works.

AM: This is the summer that I'm five years old. Preschool is behind me, and kindergarten is ahead of me. My brothers (ages two and eight) and I are chasing each other, playing tag in the backyard, all of us bare-chested, wearing shorts, wild and free. Bigbro and I agree to take turns letting Lilbro catch us and then let him get away. The sun warms my skin to a subtle pink and breezes ruffle my pageboy hairstyle as I run barefoot through the grass. Our screeching and laughter echoes off the neighboring houses but is halted by my father's voice.

"Deborah, come in and put a shirt on," he calls.

"Why? It's hot out. I don't need one." I am surprised by his request.

"Yes, you do." He insists. "Come on in, Honey. It will only take a minute, and then you can go back out and keep playing." He's not joking.

"It's too hot!" I retort. "I don't want to wear a shirt. Do Bigbro and Lilbro have to wear one?"

"No."

"Why not? If they don't have to wear one, I don't have to wear one." I cross my arms and stand my ground, determined not to give in to my dad's demand.

"Boys don't have to wear shirts," he explains, "but you're a girl and you are getting too old to run around without a shirt on anymore."

"But I've never had to wear one to just go out and play before." My lower lip juts out into a full pout.

"You're going to start kindergarten this year, and kindergarten girls always wear shirts."

"That's not fair! Just because I'm a girl, I have to wear a shirt?" I fume.

As the argument continues, I am incensed and outraged at how unfair this is. I can't believe my dad is going along with this weird girl rule and is not siding with me. It doesn't make sense. I am powerless and frustrated and hate being stuck in this girl body. "Well, if I can't play outside without a shirt on, I just won't play outside anymore!" Tears spill from my eyes as I run into the house in protest.

"That's fine, Honey, you don't have to play outside if you don't want to. But if you *do* want to play outside, make sure you put on a shirt." His words trailing after me are final.

When I reach my bedroom, I flop onto the bed, squeeze my pillow tight, and sob long and hard. I cry for my loss of freedom. I cry that boys can do whatever they want to, and girls can't. I cry for all girls everywhere, protesting aloud, "It's not fair!" My cries are inconsolable. I did not play outside again that day.

Instead, I decide to go on a play strike. If I can't play outside bare-chested like my brothers and the neighbor boys, like I always have before, then I'm not going out to play at all. Ever again. Period. My strike lasts three days. I can't keep it up, especially when Mom and Dad rule that I have to wear a shirt at all times, even indoors, too. At this point, utterly defeated, I surrender, hanging my head, donning my summer top like a shroud.

FM: *Whoops!* I accidentally let it slip. The words "Special Game," which I promised never to mention, came spilling out of my mouth in an argument with my mother. I am really mad at her. She is forbidding me to camp out in the neighbor's backyard tent with Bigbro because I'm too little. I'm sure when I ask Dad, he will say yes and let me camp with the big kids, so I ignore her and dig my sleeping bag out of the closet. She insists Dad will also say no and orders me to put my sleeping bag away. To prove to her that Dad will side with me, I blurt out, "Well, you might not let me sleep in a tent, but Dad will because he calls me his Big Girl and plays a Special Game with me. It's a secret between just me and him, and no one else can play with us, not even you!" I instantly realize my mistake and regret it, as my words echo between us.

"What game?" she interrogates me.

At first, I stay silent with a blank stare, too nervous to answer. Mom repeats the question. It is too late to take back my words, so I offer, "It's a secret, and I promised not to tell. You'll have to ask Dad. He can tell you about the game if he wants to." I have already said too much. After the argument with my mom, I am nervous about my grave mistake and about my dad coming home from work. Will she ask him about the Special Game? Or maybe she'll just forget about it, and then I won't get into trouble with Dad. I hope for the rest of the day that Mom won't mention it.

My hopes are dashed. Soon after my dad's return home, I hear my parents arguing upstairs in their bedroom, behind closed doors. I creep upstairs to my bedroom, next to theirs, so I am able to listen to what they are saying. Their voices carry loud enough that I don't have to strain to hear.

"What Special Game is Deborah talking about?" Mom demands to know.

Dad lies, sounding incredulous, "I don't know what game she's talking about! She's just a little girl with a wild imagination. It could be anything. She could be talking about Checkers for Crissake!"

As they argue, my child mind does not know that my mom is fighting to protect me, and that my dad is fighting to keep abusing me and keep himself from being exposed. Instead, I think that the Special Game makes Mom jealous, and that she wants to play, too.

It takes some finagling, but Dad successfully lies his way out of my slip-up. He seeks me out later in my bedroom when Mom is out of earshot. I think that he is going to bawl me out or perhaps even give me a spanking, but he is surprisingly calm at my profuse apology.

"I'm sorry. I didn't mean to say anything. It just slipped out."

"I know. I'm glad you didn't tell Mom anything about the game. We'll just have to stop playing it for a while," he sounds disappointed on my behalf.

I offer a solution, "We can let Mom play, too. I don't mind if she plays with us. Maybe then she won't be so mad."

He doesn't think that is a good idea but does think that we should just take a break and not play as often. That is fine by me. It never occurs to me to seek Dad out to play the Special Game anyway. When he wants to play, he always initiates it. Most times, when Mom isn't around, I try to avoid him because more and more I don't want to play. I am old enough now to leave the house on my own and seek out the neighborhood kids available to play with me. The Special Game makes me feel uncomfortable, but I can't explain why. I feel self-conscious and guarded when my dad and I touch each other. I'm glad to have a break.

AM: Midsummer of my fifth year, the shirt incident is behind me, though not forgotten. I've become accustomed to wearing tops, no matter how hot, just like the older girls on the block. They don't seem to mind it, so I try not to.

Today is another bike-riding lesson from Dad. Shady Lane is not a through street, so there are very few cars that ever drive through our neighborhood. Most cars are parked in the alley in garages behind the houses, so it is easy for the neighborhood kids to play safely in the street. It is also suitable to learn how to ride a bike here.

My bike doesn't have training wheels, and I don't want them. The fixer-upper two-wheeler my dad found in a classified ad is purple, my favorite color, with a sparkly silver banana seat. No more trying to ride Bigbro's old bike that he outgrew. Mine is better, because the frame dips down at an angle and is easier for me to get on and off. I only rolled around on my brother's old bike, gliding along, letting my straddled legs dangle on either side so I could stop myself with my feet. Now that I have a bike of my very own, it is time to learn how to pedal.

I am determined to teach myself. Pushing off the curb, I slowly pedal and wobble until both me and the bike tip over into the grassy verge. Many days of leg bruises and skinned elbows eventually lead to frustrated tears. As I weep softly, crumpled by the curb, I tell myself I don't care if I am the only kid in all of kindergarten who doesn't know how to ride a bike. And if I never learn, that is okay, too. So what if every other kid in the whole world can ride and I can't? I will live without bike riding and find other things to do.

It isn't that I don't want to learn how to ride my bike. It is just that I have tried and failed enough times on my own that I don't think I am capable of learning this particular skill. That's when Dad comes to the rescue. He says he will teach me, and with his help, he thinks I can do it. I hope he's right.

I am ready for the familiar and steady push, as my dad runs alongside me and my bike, one hand braced behind the seat, and his other hand steadying the handlebars. This time, Dad lets go, and I sail down the street alone. I am doing it! I am riding my bike and not tipping over! Dad sprints in front of me to glide me to a stop.

"Wow! Look at you! You did great!" He praises my effort.

I join in, "Did you see that, Dad? I was really riding!" My excitement pours out of me through the words, "Push me again!" I have only managed pedaling forward and have yet to master rocking the pedals backward to brake to a stop. Each time down the street now, Dad lets go, and runs ahead to catch me.

By the next training session, I am riding, turning and even braking like a pro. I just can't get started without a push.

"Try standing up when you start to pedal, rather than sitting on the seat first. You'll get more momentum that way," Dad gives me pointers. He is right. I stand up to start and wobble a bit while I strain to push the pedals one after the other. After only a few presses, I am steady and sit down as I reach cruising speed. Now it's my turn to whoop and holler!

"Woohoo! Look at me! I'm riding! I'm riding!" I smile big at the neighbor kids in their yards, watching me whoosh by them. What a relief! I am no longer the kid resigned never to be able to ride a bike. I am just like everybody else, zooming around the neighborhood on two wheels. "Thanks, Dad!"

On this triumphant day, how could either of us know that in eight years, my newfound freedom and independence would lead to a bike-riding tragedy?

*She waits under stone
'til the bridge of night
when the last blue blackens
and coats the moon.*

*Because she wakes,
you'll not rest.*

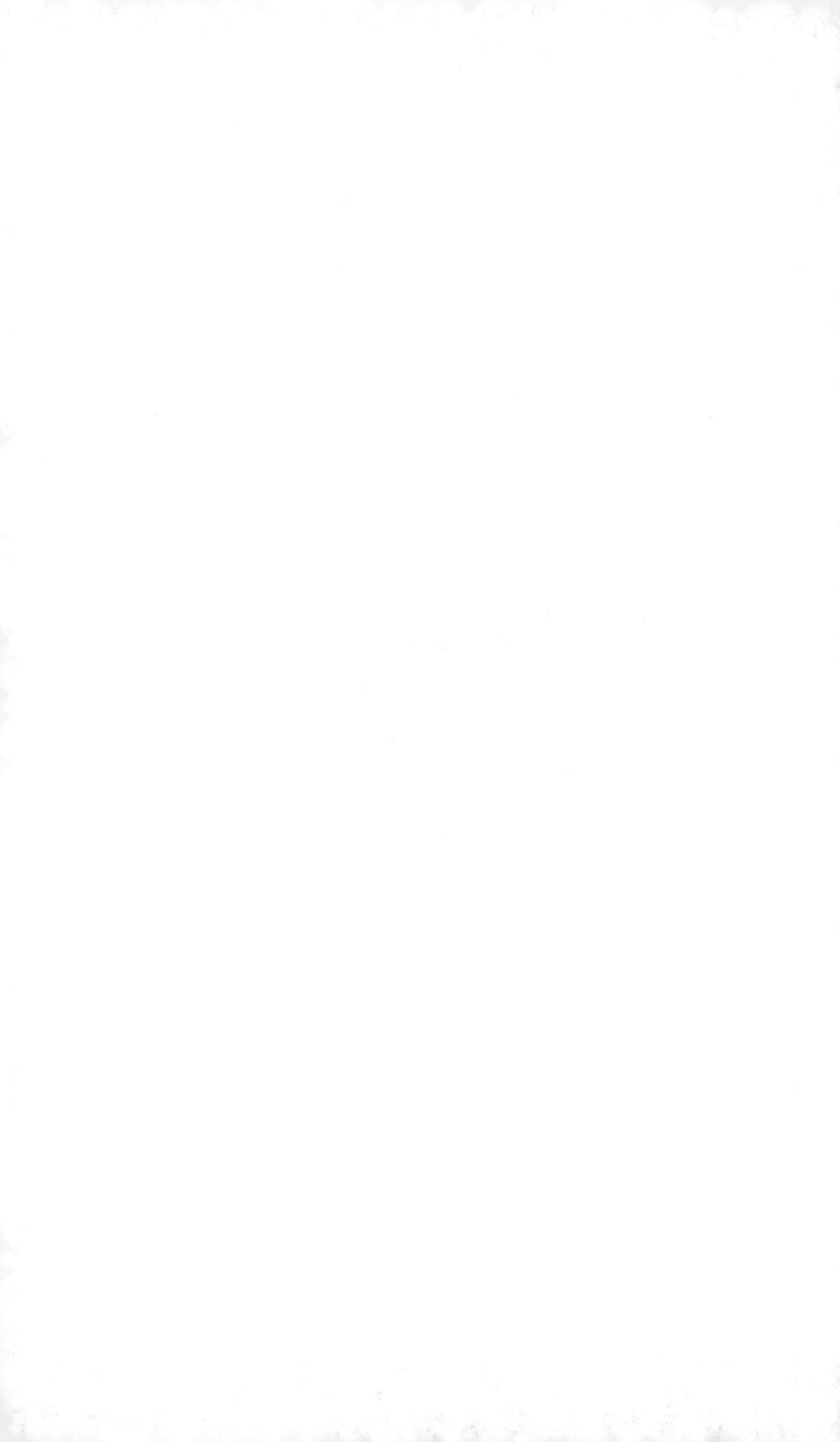

Chapter 2

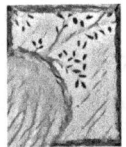

Denial is Stronger than Memory

FM: Things change suddenly and forever in the dead of night when I am seven years old. For the first time, Dad attempts to penetrate me. For the first time, the Special Game hurts, right between my legs. I cry out in pain and surprise. Mom bursts through my bedroom door, flicks the blackness into a blinding white glare, catching him in the act: my dad, in my bed, on top of me.

Pandemonium ensues. My parents' voices erupt into accusations and threats. The audio is more memorable to me than the visual, as I am blinded by the ceiling light.

"What on earth? Get off of her! What are you doing?" Mom screams.

Dad leaps out of bed and jumps into his tightywhities, pulling them up while he stammers incoherently, "It's not what you think! It's just this one time! I've never done this before!" He shifts his comments to me, "I'm so sorry, Honey. Dad didn't mean to hurt you. Are you okay? Dad's sorry!"

"I'm okay, Dad," I sniffle.

Mom shrieks, "She's not okay. Look at her! She's bleeding! We have to take her to the hospital." I glance down my legs to see drops of blood down one inner thigh that stop at my knee.

Dad retorts, "No, we can't do that! They'll take her away from us!" He shifts his talk to me again, "You don't want to live somewhere else, do you, Honey? Do you want to be taken away and never see me or Mom again?"

"No, Dad," I'm still sniffling. What in the world is he talking about? Where could I possibly be going?

"But she needs help. She's hurt. Get dressed." Mom orders both of us, "We're going to the hospital."

Dad accelerates to full panic mode, "The doctors will know what happened, and they'll call the police, and I'll be arrested and go to jail, and they'll take her away from us!"

"We're going!" Mom is undeterred.

"No, we're not!" he rants. "Where will you live with me in jail? You have no job, no money to keep the house. You'll end up living on the street. Do you want everyone to know our business? Everyone will know! We have to keep her here with us. We can clean her up. She'll be fine. We have to keep the family together!" Back to me again, "Are you okay, Sweetheart? You're okay, aren't you?"

"I think I'm okay, Dad. I don't need to go to the hospital. I don't want to go to the hospital," I decide. The swirling words of their argument frightened me more than whatever has physically happened to me. Why would there be police at the hospital? Why would Dad be arrested? Where would Mom and my brothers and I live if Dad went to jail? I don't understand why they are talking about all these things.

"You see? She says she's fine. Get a wet washcloth, and we'll fix her up," Dad begins to take charge.

I can see Mom's face fall as she relents. Her voice collapses through frustrated tears, but she still manages to threaten Dad, "If I can't get this bleeding to stop, we're leaving without you, and you'd better run! I'll give you a head start. I don't care who knows. The rest of us can live with my mother. I can get a job. We'll be fine, but will you?" She storms down the hall to the bathroom, and I hear her start the bathtub faucet. Dad's face goes white as her threat stuns him into silence.

With the water still running, she comes back with the damp washcloth. The bleeding had already stopped on its own, and there were only a few drops of blood on the bed sheet, and the drops on my leg had already dried. "Go sit in the tub," Mom tells me, and for the first time since the ordeal began, I move from lying on my back where I've remained this whole time. I'm sore in my groin as I walk with a gimpy limp down the hallway to the tub. The straddle step into the tub doesn't feel any better, but I find some comfort in the warm water as I sit, alone, in the bathroom. As soon as my bottom half is completely submerged, I turn off the faucet.

It seems bizarre to me, at both the age I am when it happened, and as an adult remembering back, that my brothers didn't wake up in all this commotion. They shared a room at the end of the hall adjacent to the bathroom, and would have been four and ten years old. Did they wake up to see what was going on and I just don't remember? Did they wake from the argument but just stay in bed? Did they sleep through the whole thing? Whatever happened then, neither of my brothers, as adults, recall this night.

Mom's voice trails down the hallway. I can hear that she is changing the sheets on my bed and still threatening my dad, "You're lucky that the bleeding stopped. This will never happen again, never!" Dad mumbles in agreement as she continues, "And we will never mention this ever again! We're all going to forget this ever happened!"

That's all I remember about that night. I don't remember getting out of the tub, or getting back in bed, or falling back to sleep. I do remember something from the next day.

Mom is in the kitchen. She is scrubbing my bed sheet from the night before in the kitchen sink that she's filled with soapy water. Most of the sheet, white with purple flowers, billows onto the floor, still dry. The top sheet and pillowcases are also crumpled on the floor. "I'm just going to get the stain out before I wash your sheets," she explains to me with a half-smile. She put the matching sheet set with pink flowers on my bed last night. I only have two sets of sheets that are designated for my bed. The white with pink roses ones are identical except in flower color to the white with purple roses ones. The part of the purple patterned sheet that now soaks in the sink has my brown blood droplets on it. No matter how much she frantically scrubs, she can't get the stains to disappear.

Eventually, she accidentally wears a hole through the sheet, which frustrates her further.

In a huff and a whirl, Mom wads the sheet into a ball, letting the water splash out of the sink and onto the floor. She scoops up the top sheet and pillowcases from the floor and wrestles the floral tangle into her arms, dripping all the while through the kitchen, out the back door and outside to the alleyway garbage cans. I trail behind her. She doesn't bother to bag up the linen refuse but tosses it, as is, into a bin and slams down the lid. The end result is that I no longer have my favorite sheets—the ones covered with purple roses.

A week or so later, it is sheet-laundering day in our house. My mom always launders all the bedsheets together, and once the beds are stripped, and the washing machine has started with the first load, she busies herself with remaking all of our beds with the fresh sheet sets from the linen closet. On this particular day I am helping her. Mom stares, blinking at the open linen closet, and then asks me, "Where are your purple sheets?" I don't know what to say to her. I watched her try to scrub them clean, tear a hole in them, and throw them away. We were both there when it happened. She continues, "I don't understand why they aren't here? Where have they gone to?"

"Don't you remember, Mom?" I try to jog her memory, "You threw them away."

"Don't be silly, Deborah. Why would I throw away a set of perfectly good sheets?"

Mom's obliviousness disturbs me. I offer further, "They had a stain you couldn't scrub out, and you tore a hole in them. That's why you threw them away. They were ruined, remember?"

She keeps blinking at me with a blank, eerie expression, as if she can't make out what I am saying.

"No, that can't be right," she seems flustered. "Are you telling me you threw your sheets away, Deborah?"

"No, Mom. I didn't throw them away. You did!" I punctuate the truth. Then I stomp off down the stairs, away from her, frustrated, mad, and confused. Really, Mom, you're going to accuse me of something that you, yourself did? Why don't you remember? I wasn't going to elaborate further about how the stain got there in the first place. It was unbelievable! Was she really so clueless?

AM: To this day, my mom doesn't recall that I was sexually abused, or the day she ended it. All these years later, Mom believes that I'm telling the truth but is baffled as to why she doesn't remember any of the scenarios that I do. I am equally baffled by her memory lapse.

I don't know exactly when my dad conveniently forgot about the Special Game, and the night Mom brought it to an explosive halt after four years. He has forgotten many things throughout his lifetime, as is his habit. For years now, in my adult life, he voluntarily admits how bad his memory is, almost like his forgetting is a badge of honor, and his memory is not getting better with age.

In my mid-40s, after a decade of mutual silence, my dad and I are on speaking terms again. Dad calls and says he's concerned that his mother, my last remaining grandparent, is going senile. She's not. Her memory has always been sharp as a tack and still is, unlike my father's.

During this crisis phone call, Dad is panicked that Grandma is inventing stories about my older brother, and Dad tells me, "She starts talking about when he played the trumpet in band in high school and she goes on about when he was in the bugle corps in the Air Force. I think she's lost it! He never played trumpet in high school, and he was never in the Air Force."

"Um... yes, Bigbro did play trumpet in high school, and, yes, he did join the Air National Guard," I tell him, and I think to myself, Grandma is not the one going senile.

"What? Are you sure? Why don't I remember that? I remember him playing trumpet in junior high, but he never played in high school marching band, did he?"

"Yes, Dad. You used to take us all to the football games to watch him march in the pregame and halftime shows, but we'd always leave the game after halftime, when the marching band show was over."

"That's what your grandma was talking about," Dad confirms and asks, "When was he in the military?"

"I don't know exactly, but don't you remember meeting him at the airport after he completed basic training? He looked all sharp in his dress blues. And he played in the bugle corps so he could march and play music instead of having to do the regular basic training drills."

"That still doesn't sound familiar to me," he hesitates.

"Why don't you call Bigbro and ask him yourself? He can tell you all about it," I recommend.

A like-father-like-son connection should have helped my dad remember these details about my older brother's life. My dad was also a trumpet player during his own school years, and my dad was a military man for a couple of years. Granted, Dad was in the Navy, not the Air Force and not the reserves, but I would think he would remember out of a sense of pride that his son followed in his footsteps, both musically and in service to our country.

Dad does call my older brother, and I hear later from Bigbro that Dad is so relieved that his mother is not senile. All the things we have said to him to confirm Grandma's memories are now starting to sound familiar to him. This supposed senility episode of my grandma's, at the time that it happened and still today, is the quintessential memory lapse of Dad's that the whole family is allowed to talk about and even joke about. Dad will even bring it up himself, "Remember when I thought my mom was going senile?" and all that are present recall and have a good laugh at my dad's expense.

As far as him not recalling the incest, Dad doesn't think the adult me is lying when I say what happened. He believes that I believe it to be true. However, he thinks I am mistaken in my memory or in identifying him as the perpetrator. He even suggests that my therapist implanted false memories in my brain, or the medications I took for bipolar disorder altered my memory. Because my dad cannot recall doing this, in his mind any details that involve him could not have happened. In a way, it is easy for me to believe my dad doesn't remember, at least not in any conscious area of his brain he can willingly access. I assume some undiagnosed mental glitch lingers within his brain somewhere. How ironic that we each assume the same about the other, that there is some medical brain anomaly that can account for the discrepancies in the events of our incompatible histories.

As for me and my forgetting, I know that by the end of my seventh summer, I have no conscious memory of the trauma that had occurred merely weeks before, or any memories of the Special Game episodes that preceded it. That's the summer we move from living in the two and a half story house in town to a ranch style house on a couple of acres of land in the countryside. That summer, the only place I have ever called home is gone, along with the bustle amidst the city streets. It seems my trauma memories were left behind in that house, in that childhood bedroom, disappearing into black hole moments of time. If only that were true. The trauma from this early time of my life settled deep within me, residing somewhere just beyond my reach.

At least my mom was right that fraught-filled night, in her orders to my dad, while I was seven and sitting in the tub. "This will never happen again, never!" It didn't. "And we will never mention this ever again!" We didn't. "We're all going to forget this ever happened!" We did.

*The faster the world spins the slower things seem
When you're trapped in a daymare
you wish were a dream.*

*I hope there's a heaven, 'cuz I visited hell.
The way ain't paved with good intentions.*

CHAPTER 3

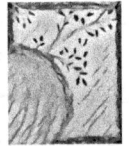

JOYRIDE

AM: "Who on this bus is only 13?" The corn detasseling supervisor scours our teenage faces with her probing eyes, as she paces up and down the center aisle of the school bus. A few brunette curls escape her ponytail and cling to her sunburned face, damp with sweat from being in the cornfields all day. She looks down her narrow nose, using it like a pointer to detect any guilty-looking expressions that will give the offending 13-year-olds away. I am one of them, with my own blonde and damp ponytail, avoiding her scrutinizing gaze. The supervisor's build is wiry but strong. She could easily brawl with someone twice her size and win. No one wants to cross her. Besides, at the moment, she is already cross enough. We all sit stock still in two rows of padded brown bench seats that run the length of the aisle as she continues to bark her interrogation, singling people out. "How old are you?" Everyone pointed to answers 14, 15, or 16. Thank God she didn't point at me. All of us teenagers know that there are at least a dozen or more who are only 13 and who they are, but no one says a word. No one wants to be a tattletale or be fired for admitting they are too young to be on the corn detasseling crew.

The problem is that the field recruiter man, who hired all of us over the phone, said it was okay to be 13. You just couldn't be 12, or he would get into trouble. You could be 13 as long as you turned 14 before the end of the year. I was 13 that summer and had a December birthday. Based on the recruiter's hiring criteria, I qualified, so I signed up. This outburst by the crew supervisor was the first I—or any of us—knew that it wasn't true.

Bigbro says I will hate detasseling. He only lasted two days the summer he tried it and now says I won't last a day. I want to outlast his two-day record for bragging rights. I also have my earnings already spent in my head. If I can make it a week, I'll have enough money to buy a 10-speed bike, a boombox, and the pair of Nike sneakers I covet. I have never owned shoes with a popular name brand before unless it came to me as a hand-me-down. I am determined to detassel the whole week to purchase my prize possessions. If I end up liking it, I can work the whole summer and feel like I've won the Publishers Clearinghouse Sweepstakes… or my 13-year-old equivalent—over a thousand dollars. Fortunately, no 13-year-olds are outed on the bus that first day.

It turns out, Bigbro is right, at least partially. I do hate detasseling. Either I am too short, or the corn is too tall. I need to get up at 4:30 a.m. to catch the bus at 5:00 a.m., and then ride half-asleep at least 45 minutes to the farm field they want us to work in that day.

First thing in the morning, the corn is damp with dew, and the leaves cling to my shirt as I walk the rows, soaking my shirt through. By early afternoon, when we quit for the day, I am still soaked, but from sweat instead of dew. It is hard to discern if the pink on my skin is more corn rash or sunburn since both patchwork my arms and face.

Wednesday is the worst day. It pours down rain, and we work anyway. The supervisor warns us all ahead of time to always be prepared, in case it rains, by bringing a trash bag to wear over our clothes like a poncho, a rain hat, and bread sacks to tie over our shoes. I would have felt self-conscious sporting this outfit alone and anywhere else, but we crew members all look the same in our goofy yet functional uniforms. The steady downpour turns muddy rows into mire, and then the mire into near quicksand. The ground suctions my feet, each step making a loud *slurp*! I can barely keep my shoes on, but with heavy marching steps manage to do so. Fortunately, after a couple of hours, thunder rumbles in the distance, and lightning streaks across the sky, which means everybody runs to the bus for shelter until the storm passes.

I'm glad it only rained one day that week, or I might not have accomplished my goal of six workdays in a row. Bigbro is impressed. He didn't think I'd make it. A few years later, Lilbro puts us both to shame, lasting over a month and now owns the bragging rights over his older siblings. As for me, I am victorious and relish my spoils. Yes, I get my boombox with the portable handle that plays cassette tapes and has a radio. Yes, I get my Nike tennis shoes, white with the red, signature swoosh emblem on both sides. And yes, I get a 10-speed Huffy Omni bike—aqua blue, shiny and new.

The bike is the biggest deal. I have long since outgrown the secondhand, purple two-wheeler with the silver banana seat that my dad taught me to ride in the old neighborhood. I've been using my mom's red three-speed—that might be from the 1950s—in the meantime. I don't know when she got it, but it seems to be an antique and is slightly too big for me. I manage to ride it anyway because of the lady's frame that angles down between the seat and the handlebars, but I can't sit on the seat with both of my feet touching the ground, not even on my tiptoes. I need to tilt one way or the other to catch myself from tipping over when I slow to a stop.

Not only is my bike brand new, but I am also the one who pays for it with my own money, so the bike is truly mine. My biggest challenge will be to see if I can get up the steep, half-mile hill that stands between me and anywhere I want to go without getting off my bike and pushing it. With my former two-wheelers, I could only make it halfway before dismounting to walk it over the top. Surely, my ten-speed in first gear will allow me to make it all the way up. After getting dropped at the store, I wheel the bike (the style I had selected weeks before) to the checkout, relieved that they still have my style and one in my size. And I get a bike lock. I wheel it outside, ready to take it on its maiden voyage.

Three miles separate the store from home. I beam as I pedal the first mile through the neighborhoods that lead to the "Winding road next 2 miles" sign, where the city streets flow into the countryside. I can pedal with ease the rise and fall of the curvy road by shifting gears up or down as needed. Another mile goes by. As I approach the fork in the road holding the "Bluffs Park 1 mile" sign with an arrow to the left, I see my challenge rise before me to the right. I'm not going to the park but rather turning upward toward home. Whether leaving home or returning, the great hill looms. In this direction, heading north, the grade is steeper, but the hill is shorter. I am determined to conquer it on wheels, not on foot.

I manage to ascend halfway using fifth gear before my pedaling slows and becomes labored. A couple more shifts to third, and I'm three-quarters of the way to the top. Second gear kicks in. Can I make it? Not quite. First gear is all I have left. I'm so close and pedaling in slow motion. I start to weave back and forth to make the last of the climb less steep... maybe if I stand up on the pedals and give a few... more... pumps... yes! I did it! I made it to the top without stopping! "Woohoo!" I voice my triumph legato and loud. My instant reward is the long downward slope to home. I shift up through the gears to tenth as I coast, picking up speed. I have enough momentum to roll into the driveway without another stroke of the pedals, never mind the last bit of lift in the road. Breathless and elated, I can't wait to tell my family that I did it. My new bike and I conquered the hill!

FM: It's a sunny summer Saturday. The country road winds four miles, door to door, to my friend Lenee's house. Lenee and I became friends when she switched to my class to start the fourth grade. I know her from our bus route over the previous years, but come to really know and like her when we spend all day in school together, grouped in the same subject-learning pods. She plays saxophone in band and outruns the boys, so she is always the first girl to get picked when we divide into playground teams. Because of our shared bus route, we moved to Cooper Junior High together. The summer between seventh and eighth grades, Lenee has yet to see my new wheels, and I am eager to show them off, as eager as I am to ride my bike and to see her again. With school out of session, friend visits are few and far between. We agree to eat lunch at her house and then spend the rest of the afternoon together. I can't wait. Today I wear my new lavender knit shorts, a matching T-shirt top, and tube socks with three parallel lavender stripes just below the knee. I tie on my Nike tennis shoes, which Lenee also has yet to see, and head out the garage door with my still shiny, still new 10-speed.

    My bike and I conquer the hill again, this time heading south, and coast around the fork, doubling back towards Bluffs Park. Once I get to the park entrance, I'll be halfway there, and then I'll hang a left off of the pavement and onto Lenee's gravel road for the remaining two miles. So far, I'm midway to the park.

    Here comes a dark, rusted out pickup truck, blaring country music, which adds to the noise of an unmuffled exhaust pipe. As the rumbling vehicle approaches me in the oncoming lane, I try to make out, is the truck black, or is it blue? It's so dirt-caked I can't tell. The three boys in the cab hang out the open windows, whistle and whoop, "Hey, Baby! Looking good!" I'm flattered that boys, old enough to drive, would pay any attention to me. I might have been okay if I had ignored them, but that's not what I do. I give them a broad smile and a two-handed wave, balancing as I cruise without using the handlebars. Pleased with myself, I keep pedaling hands-free as they zoom past me, giving me a few horn honks and hollers. I don't recognize these boys. The Texas license plates make me assume they are on vacation, here to visit someone local. I wish this was the end of the story. I wish I could meet up with my friend, Lenee, and impishly tell her the story of the older Texas teens noticing me. But no.

I hear tires squeal from behind. A quick backward glance tells me the truck made a tight U-turn, and the rumbling hootenanny crescendos as it catches up with me.

"Just keep pedaling," I tell myself. My hands return firmly to the handlebars now. "Why on earth did I wave?" I mutter. The hairs on my neck spike as they roar up and swerve around me.

Maybe they'll just keep going, back to the park where they came from. Wishful thinking. I see them do a donut at the park entrance and head back towards me. Another boisterous drive-by and another burning rubber U-turn squeals from behind. I pray for them to go away, but this time I hear the engine slow to a sputter as they sidle in beside my bike, truck wheels rolling even with my 10-speed pedal strokes. My former flashy grin wanes to a nervous, barely-there smile, politeness masking fear.

The driver leans across his two buddies, "Need a lift?"

"Nah, I'm not going far," I decline and focus my attention on reaching the halfway point at the park entrance in front of me. Nearly there.

"Where ya goin'?" The engine sputters alongside, still matching my pace. I glance over. The driver looks and sounds more like Cary Grant than the Big Bad Wolf. I relax a bit, noticing that the trio looks to be about Bigbro's age or a little older. Maybe the locals they are in town to visit are one of my brother's buddies.

"Just to a friend's house, down the road apiece." I point one-handed to the south fork that changes from blacktop into gravel, heading away from the park.

"Well, let us take you," he says with a wry smile. "You and your bike can hop in the back," his thumb indicates the truck bed, "and we'll drop you off."

It would be nice to avoid maneuvering my thin tires in the shifting gravel as I turn onto Lenee's road for the remaining two-mile stretch. I sheepishly agree, partly because my rolling chat with the driver has eased my flight senses, and partly because I am afraid to offend the three of them by declining their kind offer.

I break to a halt, sidestep my bike, and start to hoist it up over the wheel well.

"Get out and help her, Dwayne," the would-be Cary Grant barks, as he pronounces "Du-Wain" with two syllables. The chubby guy with the dishwater blond bowl cut nearest the passenger door exits the cab. The door creaks as if it will fall off the hinges, and he leaves it dangling open as he lumbers over to me.

"Here, give me the bike," he says. His voice is a breathy, whiny falsetto. Not what I was expecting from a big guy. "You jump in the bed, and I'll hand it to you."

"Thanks," I reply, noting how easily he grabs my bike and flings it around. I hope he doesn't scratch the paint on the metal edge of the truck bed. I scale over the wheel well and then steady my stance, standing at the ready in the bed of the truck. As I reach out my arms to retrieve the bike, the person called Dwayne thrusts my bike into my chest like a battering ram, knocking me back off my feet. I land hard with a thud, butt first on metal ridges, and see my bike sailing midair into the grassy ditch. Dwayne jumps in the cab, yelling, "Go, go, go! We got her!"

The pickup tires squeal as if peeling away from a crime scene. I try to right myself, but the erratic driver veers in zigzags and keeps me tumbling precariously in the open carriage. I grasp the metal edge with both hands and peer over at the pavement speeding by. The truck is zooming too fast for me to jump. I look up through the rear cab window and on through the windshield. They're heading into the park. My mind panics at the thought of being taken across state lines. "I'm being kidnapped!" I think. The other park entrance is close to two other state borders. I worry that if they drive me across state lines, I might never see my family again. My God, are they taking me to Texas?

My brain swirls, trying to rapidly translate what is happening. Okay, don't panic. The next time they slow down, just jump and run. I catch the face of the middle guy staring back at me. He looks terrified. I'm not sure why. I'm the one being kidnapped, not him. I hear incoherent words flying out the open windows that sound like an argument. I strain to hear what they are saying but can't. Between the music and the muffler and the wind whooshing past my ears, any attempts to decipher their banter is useless. I repeat my plan, "Jump and run, jump and run. When they slow down, just jump and run."

Slowing down comes sooner than I think. Why did they pull into a dead-end overlook? No time to wonder. Jump and run! I do, dashing back towards the main road in an adrenaline sprint.

"Gus, she's getting away," Dwayne's voice screeches.

Another voice cracks, "Just let her go! I don't want to. Not like this!" It must be the middle seat guy, the one who looked terrified, staring back at me through the back window as I was trapped in the swerving, open cage.

My escape doesn't last long. The driver, Cary Grant, otherwise known as Gus, easily overtakes me saying, "Oh, no you don't! Where do you think you're going?" as he grabs me around the waist from behind. He plucks me off of my feet with one arm as easily as picking up a rag doll.

I thrash about to no avail, "Let me go!"

"I don't think so. Not until we're done with you."

What on earth does that mean? Are they going to beat me up? He heads back toward the truck, me still a struggling tangle in his arm. One of my kicks strikes with force, square on Gus's shin.

"Owww!" he grimaces. I turn to look, and he strikes me hard across the face, "Dumb bitch!" The pain blinds me. Even as my eyelids close, I see stars. It doesn't sting, it hurts. My cheek and jaw feel like I've been hit by a brick. Was that the back of his hand, or his fist that hit me? Either way, I am instantly shocked into silence and stillness. I fall limp in his grasp, stunned like a bird that smacks into a plate glass window.

Gus carries me a ways in front of the truck and throws me to the ground. No one can see us from the main road. Where are the other cars? Where are the other people? It's a gorgeous Saturday in the park. How is it that we find ourselves alone? It's broad daylight! I curl into a fetal position on the ground and brace for more blows that are sure to come, but there are none.

Instead, I'm forced spread-eagle onto my back. "Hold down her arms," Gus orders, and Dwayne pulls my arms above my head and kneels, one knee on each of my arms. Gus yanks my shirt up to my neck, along with my training bra, exposing my nipples. "Well, what do we have here?" he says, brushing my breasts. "You don't even have your boobies yet. They're barely mosquito bites." He laughs, seemingly amused with himself, and Dwayne chuckles along. I just lay there, somehow knowing and yet not knowing what will come next. Gus yanks down my shorts, wriggles them off over my shoes, and casts them aside. He does the same with my panties. I don't fight him. He leaves my shoes and socks intact. I am lying there, pinned at the arms, naked from neck to knee. "Come on, Carl, she's ready and waiting for you," Gus sneers.

I turn my head to the left to see the boy named Carl leaning with his back against a tree. He's anxiously shifting his feet from side to side, like a tyke who urgently needs to pee. Cradling his head in one elbow, hiding his eyes, he sniffles. "I told you, I don't want to anymore. Can't we just let her go?"

Yes, I think, and hold out hope that he will convince his crime partners to set me free. Carl's face twists in anguish, dotted in red spots that match his flattop buzz cut. I can't make out which dots are freckles and which dots are acne. I feel sorry for him. He regrets his choice in friends as much as I do.

"Relax, Carl. I'll warm her up for you. Let me show you how it's done." Gus knee straddles over me, unzips his jeans and lowers them just enough to jam his cock between my legs. It burns like fire. I cry out involuntarily. "Cover her mouth to shut her up," he yells. I'm not crying out for help; I'm crying out in pain. Dwayne's heavy, sweaty palm muffles my cries. I can feel gravel digging into my back with each thrust. I have no words to describe what he's doing. Suddenly, a phantom voice within me says, "Here we go again."

I drift out of my body before Gus finishes. Part of me now floats above the scene, seeing and hearing everything happening below from a satellite view, as if I'm watching a movie, as if the attack is happening to someone else.

Voices drift up from below, "There you go, Buddy Boy. That's how you do it." Gus gets up from his knees, sidesteps me, and reassembles his pants. "Are you ready to become a man?" Carl doesn't move. I'm still pinned but no longer hand gagged. "What's the matter, Carl. Can't get it up? Just rub your dick. It will get hard." Carl, still up against the tree, is visibly crying now. "Why are you crying, Carl? This is all your fault. We're doing this for you. You can't stay a virgin the rest of your life. We paid that girl from school to screw you and she refused, so we nabbed this one for you. You're too ugly to get a girl any other way. Now's your chance, Carl. Be a man!"

Carl, sobbing now, makes a beeline for the truck cab, gets in and shouts, "Fuck you!" as the door slams shut.

Gus just laughs, "No, fuck you, Carl. That's the whole point." He sidebars to Dwyane, "Can you believe it? After all we do for him, he's not even going to go through with it." Back at Carl, "You're going to be a virgin forever!"

Dwayne chuckles, "Maybe he's gay."

Gus runs with Dwayne's comment, "That's it, isn't it? Are you gay, Carl? Is that why you won't fuck her? Jeezus, Carl, you could have told us that sooner. We would have gotten you a boy instead."

"I'm not gay!" Carl hollers back and cries harder.

Gus says to Dwayne, "I guess it's your turn, if you want to."

Dwayne eagerly switches places. My numb body no longer feels anything. The me that's looking down sees the me lying on the ground staring blankly into the sky. The me on the ground notices to herself, "The sky is a beautiful shade of blue, and the clouds look like billowing cotton candy. The sunshine feels warm on my face. I can smell a hint of sweet grasses in the breeze. This is an otherwise perfect day."

Dwayne's mount takes longer, his breathing much heavier, more like wheezing. He ends with a grunt, still falsetto. When Dwayne finally gets off me, he struts back to the truck. Before Gus goes away, he stands with one foot pushing the middle of my chest and says, "Now repeat after me, 'Nothing happened.' Say it!" He demands of me. "Say it! Say 'Nothing happened.'"

My voice is but a choked whisper, "Nothing happened."

"I can't hear you. Say it so I can hear you. 'Nothing happened.'"

I clear my throat, "Nothing happened."

"That's right. When someone asks you what happened, you say, 'Nothing happened.' What happened?"

"Nothing happened." I parrot.

"Now we're going to pull out of here, but you're going to lay here and not move until you count to a hundred." His foot is still on my chest. "If you stop counting, I'll know, and I'll come back here. But if you count to a hundred, you're free to go. Let me hear you count."

"One, two, three,…" I continue.

He walks away and calls back, "Keep counting, that's good, don't stop, all the way to a hundred."

"…eleven, twelve, thirteen,…"

The pickup truck starts with a jarring blast of the muffler and music. I hear the gravel crunch and wait for the roar to fade away.

"…twenty-three, twenty-four, twenty-five." I stop counting. I need to get out of here and fast.

I roll to my stomach, relieved to look up and see that the truck and the three boys are really gone. Survival mode kicks in. I stand up and pull my bra and shirt back down, re-covering my torso. Where are my panties? They are dangling on a brush twig. Retrieve them. Put them on. I step awkwardly through the leg holes with my shoes on. Where are my shorts? Draped over a plume of grass. Retrieve them. Put them on. It is even more awkward to step through the leg holes of my shorts with my shoes on, but I manage to without falling down.

Which way do I go? My breath is audible, shallow, and quick. I need to crest the hill beside me to see where I am. I run through the tall grass, up the hill, crouching as I go so as not to be seen. There is no path. I make my own and ignore the brush's snags and scratches. Atop the hill, I see down to where the marked horse trail leads out of the park and back onto the parking area adjacent to the park entrance road. This is where I would have turned onto the gravel road to go to Lenee's house. I now know where I am.

The grassy embankment above the horse trail is steep. I leap sideways, feet first, a long slide to the ground below. Reaching the bottom, I scan my surroundings. No one is in view, but I hear horse hooves clopping and people's voices in the air. I wait, relieved that these sounds are fading away from me, not heading in my direction. All clear, I sprint the length of the horse trail ravine and race up the last hillcrest to the parking lot, panting the whole way. I reach the top and duck behind a tree, peering around its trunk. There is one empty horse trailer attached to a fancy pickup and two other cars. Thankfully, all are vacant.

Now the tricky part. I don't want to follow along the road. What if those jerks are still driving around and see me? From where I am, I still have to cross roads twice: first this gravel one beyond the parking lot that I would have taken to Lenee's house; and then, after cutting through the corner hayfield, the road I was originally snatched from. Crossing there, I can keep to the fields, over two hills and five properties to the ravine behind my house. My only choice is to go for it.

Alertness peaked, I scan my surroundings. All clear. I sprint across the parking lot and the gravel road and disappear into the ditch on the other side. After sliding under the barbed wire fence, I hustle my way through the hayfield to the paved road ditch just beyond. I crouch in the ditch, peeking just above it to make sure no one is coming. Two cars are heading this way, but not the loud, junky truck. I duck down until they pass. All clear. I scurry to the ditch on the opposite roadside. My bike! Here's my bike. I can't ride it home right now. I'm too scared to ride along the road with those awful guys driving around God knows where, and I can't take it with me cross country, but I can hide it in the longer grass so no one can see it. I don't want it to get stolen. I position my bike, concealing it just so, and note the nearest mailbox—"Thompson." A boy in my grade lives there. I'll come get the bike later.

I hope people don't notice me wandering through their properties. After scaling the first hill of the Thompson farm, I am no longer worried about being spotted by my attackers, but I am still breathless and scanning to keep out of sight. I just want to get home as fast as possible. But what will I tell my parents?

Something inside me warns me not to tell them what has just happened. That something I buried long ago but I can't quite reach—that something that still has influence over me, that forgotten history—knows my parents are not safe to trust. I cannot tell them or anyone about this assault. It feels right to hide it, to bury it. Besides, things like this are to be forgotten and never spoken of again, right?

Why does that seem to be true? I don't know, but I know that this attack is a secret I shouldn't talk about and should just forget about. In order to do that, I have to concoct a believable tale as to why I didn't go to Lenee's house and why my bike is in a ditch. Scenarios, one after the other, sift through my brain, like I am the dealer and the player in a card game, gambling on my fate, discarding, shuffling, and redealing until I have a hand that I can play. A believable lie shifts into place.

I'm riding my bike to Lenee's house when suddenly I feel ill. I'm too sick to keep going, so I turn around to head back home. I'm so dizzy, it's easier to get off and push my bike home instead. A friend of Bigbro drives past me, sees me pushing my bike and asks if I need help. He offers me a ride home but can't fit my bike into the trunk of his yellow Beetle car. I tell my brother's friend that we can hide my bike in the ditch, so it won't get stolen, and my dad and I can retrieve it later with Dad's pickup truck. Bigbro's friend drives me home, end of story. It is the best fib I can come up with, so it has to work. No one is supposed to be at home right now. The house should be empty. If that is so, the lie will work. I pray all is as it should be and that no one is at home when I arrive. When I see that our family cars are gone, I breathe a sigh of relief. The house will be empty.

My heightened vigilance disappears once I am certain I am alone and safely through the door of my home. My back leans against the safe, sealed barrier, and I collapse, sliding down the door into a sobbing pile on the floor. The pain I have been blocking—from the face smack, back gravel, and burning groin—returns. Mid-sob, a wave of nausea hits me, and I run to the bathroom just in time to vomit into the toilet. I flush the stool and sit next to it on the floor and keep crying, the sound of my sobs bouncing off the tiled wall for longer than I would ever have thought possible. My mind can't make sense of what has happened. I feel gross and dirty from the inside out. I need to wash this all away. Still crying, I fill the bathtub, strip down, and get in. I can't wash myself fast enough or vigorously enough, but once I've done a thorough cleaning from head to toe twice, I just sit and sob some more.

The tears finally subside. Now I am still, sitting in the tub, silent and staring. All I feel is numb. It's a familiar numbness that I know well, but I cannot place its origin. At some point, I exit the tub, as the water is long cold, and go into a strange autopilot.

I pull fresh clothes over my skin. My lavender outfit, strewn dirty on the floor, I know I must throw away. All of it. I can't let the pieces lie in the garbage can, or someone might see them and ask me why I threw away my perfectly good clothes. I hide the tainted garments in a paper grocery sack. Shorts, undies, top, and favorite socks, all go into the bag. Then, curling the top down and rolling it tight, I throw the bag away. I don't know why, but it's the right thing to do.

I would throw away my tennis shoes too, but I can't. My parents would obviously notice my new Nike shoes missing, and no lie would be clever enough to explain them away. I take the contraband to the outdoor garbage cans. Finding a bin that is already full, I dump out the contents, conceal my bagged evidence in the bottom of the bin, and rearrange the refuse to cover my stash. There! No one will ever know I have thrown my clothes away.

Reentering the house, it dawns on me that I need to call Lenee and explain why I never showed up. *Gasp!* Look at the time. It's almost one o'clock! I was supposed to arrive an hour and a half ago. I take a deep breath and dial her number.

Lenee can tell from my voice that something is wrong and asks what it is. "Nothing, I just don't feel well." I spin my lie, "I got sick on the way to your house and had to turn around and come home." It's hard to speak, and my voice is scratchy from crying and retching. "I was so tired and dizzy when I got home, I laid down and fell asleep. I'm so sorry I didn't call you sooner, but I just woke up." Lenee sounds relieved but needs a few more reassurances that I am okay. With a click of the receiver, the phone call ends, and I can lie down for real. I choose the couch.

As I lie on the couch, the details of my fresh assault become fuzzy and begin to fade. The sights, sounds, and sensations dissipate into an unreal dream. "Nothing happened," I repeat to myself, until I, too, believe this lie to be true. The whole event disappears out of sight, out of sound, out of feeling, and goes who knows where? Another moment vanishes into the black hole.

My cover story becomes the predominant voice in my head, and I can visualize everything I invented really happening. I replay it in my mind until I've got it memorized. By the time my parents arrive home an hour later, the attack has been erased completely from my conscious mind. I don't worry that they won't believe me, because I believe me, and I can no longer retrieve the backstory that necessitated the lie. Besides, I look and feel ghastly.

AM: Bigbro wants to talk to me. We're both standing in the front yard of our ranch house along the road. I have just returned from somewhere with my bike in tow. He sounds serious and says to me, "The other day, you told Mom and Dad that my friend gave you a ride home from the road when you were feeling sick."

"Yeah…," I recall the scenario, hesitating, feeling a bit numb and nervous, but not knowing why.

"I thanked my friend for looking out for you, and he had no idea what I was talking about. He says he didn't give you a ride, not then or any other time."

"Well, he did," I insist. "I don't know why he would lie to you about that."

"The thing is, I don't think he's lying." My brother looks at me as if I should fess up to something.

"Well, he is lying because I'm not!" I stomp away, wheeling my bike to the garage, angry and confused. Did I lie? No. Yes. No. Yes. No. My mind is a blur between true and false. Why would my brother's friend say he didn't give me a ride when he did? Doesn't he want the credit for doing a good deed and rescuing me? None of this makes any sense.

AM: It's day one of eighth grade, after my first teenage summer. I can ride my new bike to school if I want to, but I decide not to, not on the first day, anyway. The school bus route has changed again, and instead of getting picked up at our front door, we have to walk to West Bend Street. It's a winding dirt side street a few lanes down the road from our lane with no outlet, and here's where we now are to wait to catch the bus. All the country kids from our area are to meet here at the one pick-up and drop-off point. This year, the route also runs clockwise to the north, not counter-clockwise as before, which means that, instead of being first on in the morning and last off in the afternoon, we are last on in the morning and first off in the afternoon. The bus will already be mostly full by the time we get on in the morning for the start of the school year. My friend Jodie and I chat casually until the bus arrives. We agree to sit together, as usual, if there is an empty seat for us to share.

When my family first moved to the acreage house six years previously, Jodie was my first and fast friend. Looking back to our introductory encounter, I remember it is summer, and I am bored playing with just my brothers all the time. In the old neighborhood we had lots of kids to pal around with, but here I don't know anybody else. The houses are blocks apart, and most are hidden away from the main road with long lanes. A retired couple lives in the only home we can see from our property. Mom tells me to walk to the next house beyond, to the driveway on the opposite side of the road and knock on the door. She says there are lots of kids in that house. She knows because she bought some fresh cream from the mom who lives there. Maybe there will be someone my age to play with.

So, my seven-year-old-self heads down the road, walking on the grassy shoulder, winding up the long gravel driveway, and to one of the doors of a big farmhouse. Is it the front door? Is it the back door? I don't know. I can't tell. When I knock, the mom answers, and I tell her where I live, and that my mom sent me here to ask her if she has any kids my age that can play with me.

The mom has a kind, grandma face, surrounded in soft brunette curls. She looks as if I caught her in the middle of something. She wipes her hands on her apron and, after looking me up and down, she calls into the house over her shoulder, "Lucy! Come here. There's someone here to meet you!"

A little girl with blonde, curly pigtails steps out of the house and walks over to me. She doesn't look very old. I tell her my name, and ask her how old she is. Turns out she's only three, a year younger than Lilbro. I ask her if there are any older kids in the house and tell her that I am seven. She eagerly goes back into the house and brings back her next oldest sister, Jodie.

Jodie is instantly my new best friend. She freely smiles and easily chats. Her long, soft and brunette hair matches her mother's. We immediately bond, laughing that her mom sent Lucy out to play with me, thinking the three-year-old Lucy and the seven-year-old me were the same age. To us the mistake is obvious, and we laugh freely about it until our sides ache. From now on and for the rest of the summer, Jodie and I will play together, climbing apple trees, running through the grassy hillsides, picking fresh corn from her father's fields, playing dolls inside on rainy days. At the end of that first summer, I am disappointed that, even though Jodie and I are both starting second grade at Parkview Elementary School, we won't have the same teacher and will be in different classrooms. Still, we will ride the bus together before and after school each day and will continue playing together outside of school hours.

Jodie and I never wind up in the same class in elementary school, but, in fifth grade, we both signed up to play clarinet in band. From that point on, from fifth grade through twelfth, we have clarinet lessons together with the band teacher, Mrs. Drake, and always sit next to each other, playing the first clarinet music part in band.

So here we are, Jodie and I, just before starting the eighth grade, waiting to see if there will be an empty seat on the bus for us to sit together. There is. The one open spot is fourth on the left as we enter. Jodie climbs in ahead of me. I hesitate. An older teen with a smirky grin is seated just behind the bench Jodie grabs for us. He's a new boy and rests his arms outstretched on his seat back, positioning himself in the middle, all casual-like. He looks like Cary Grant and stares right through me, knowingly. I meet his gaze. A visceral knot of fear tightens my stomach. My cheeks go pale as he continues to smirk and stare and then gives me a wink.

I flinch. I must look dazed because Jodie then says, "Do you know him?" as she motions for me to sit down and glances back at him. I'm holding up the line of kids behind me.

"Down in front," I hear someone call from behind, and another kid's voice says, "Yah, sit down."

I sit and can feel Cary Grant's eyeballs boring two holes in the back of my head.

"I've never seen him before in my life," I tell Jodie, in hushed tones. "He just looks like someone else I used to know and didn't like, but I can't place him."

After a few bus rides and rounds of chatter and gossip amongst the bus kids, it turns out the new guy is from Texas and is a high school cousin of a pair of sisters on our route. He is living with them temporarily. Gus got in trouble back home in Austin for hot-wiring cars and flunking out of school and is now staying with his aunt and uncle on the farm to try to get him straightened out. He sports the posture of a cocky troublemaker, with a mocking mouth to match. Before long, Gus is missing from the bus. Rumor has it, he got sent to reform school, or back to Texas, or was maybe even arrested and thrown in jail, depending on who you asked. He joined us on the bus just briefly, a month into the semester, and then was gone.

I do—later, in all my adult rememberings—recall that the new boy on the bus that fall was the ringleader rapist. I have no doubt. If I—as an adult—wanted to find him, I'm sure I could track him down to see whatever became of him by finding his cousins online and surfing the internet. I don't want to seek him out.

I have no desire to dredge him up. I'd rather Gus, or Cary Grant, or whoever he is, stay in the past where he belongs, away from me, gone forever.

AM: "Mom," I call out, unable to find the socks I am looking for, "have you seen my favorite tube socks, the ones with the three lavender stripes?" No, she has no idea where they are. I had two like pairs, one with purple stripes and one with pink stripes. I often wonder when wearing my pinked striped pair, whatever happened to my matching white tube socks with the purple stripes? It's like they just disappeared.

*A cold, dark room
full of shadows,
the door locked
from the outside.*

Nothing can escape.

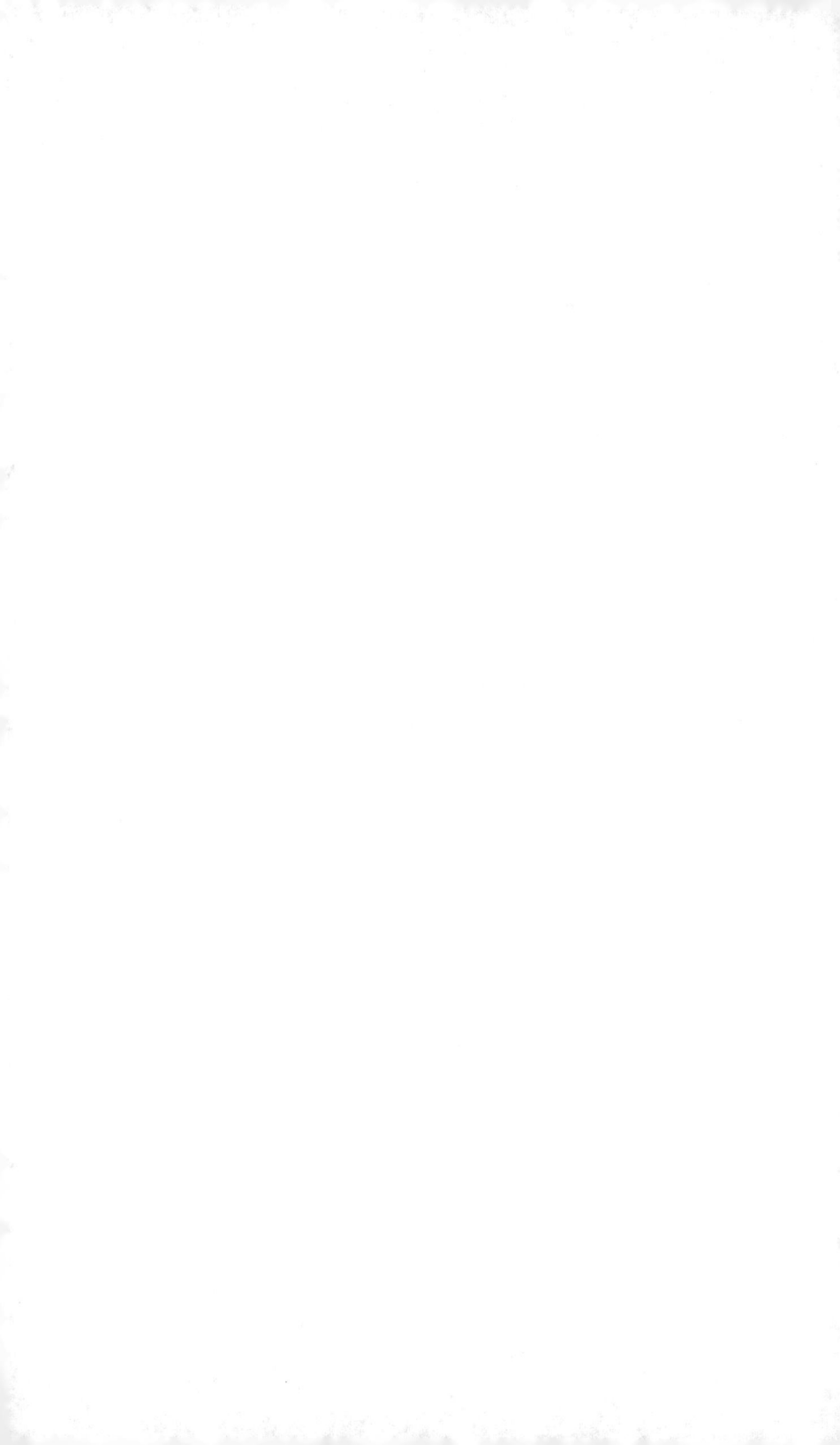

Chapter 4

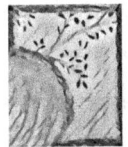

The Shadow Monster

If my hindsight is 20/20, like everyone else's, here is what I see clearly as my fully remembering adult self looks back over my childhood. As a child, my survival depended on my parents. I had no control over the decisions they made or the environment they created. Without power or choice, I adapted. My parents decided we would never talk about the night my mom entered my bedroom, exposing Dad's unholy act, and they went on as if nothing had happened. I just followed their lead. But not talking about the damage did not make it go away. Forgetting about the damage did not make it go away. I remained damaged.

So, the damaged version of me splintered off, needing to become separate within my subconscious mind. She peeled herself from me as if I were dividing into two identical cells. Twins. Except the new twin was frozen in space, frozen in pain, frozen in fear, frozen at the core, while the rest of me—the forgetting twin—carried on as if nothing had happened. The frozen twin was at the same time ages seven, six, five, four, and three, like nesting dolls, holding all of the incest memories, up through Dad's final act. She was locked in a room, wounded, scared, and alone, left to fend for herself. We were one in the same, I was her jailer, and she was my prisoner; I didn't remember her, but she remembered me, and she didn't forget, even though I did.

The damaged part of me from the rape splintered in the same way, burrowing in to hide in my subconscious. Now there were two wounded captives within me: the three-to-seven-year-old child incest victim, who already resided in her prison cell, and the new arrival, the thirteen-year-old teenager rape victim. I locked them in adjoining cells. They could hear each other but couldn't see each other. Neither captive was aware that they were, in fact, clones of each other and of their jailer. The jailer—me—was clueless. I had no idea these prisoner twins of me existed, that they had split off within my subconscious, that they had survived, and that they were working full-time to be recognized. I functioned in oblivious autopilot, though occasionally had a fleeting thought and wondered, "Why do I feel less happy than my friends do? Their happiness seems genuine." I'm just role-playing "happy" to fit in.

Not remembering either trauma was essential to surviving my daily childhood life and continued into adulthood. To accomplish this, I had to keep any awareness or sense of trauma out of my conscious mind. I felt something was off, but I was unaware there were parts of me I couldn't reach, parts that were screaming to be heard, screaming to be set free, screaming to be healed.

What I consciously experienced during the era I was aged 7 to 29, the years when I sufficiently blocked out the buried trauma, was a dark, nebulous murkiness within, a heaviness I carried wherever I went. I tried to ignore it, but it was always with me. I felt its eerie presence. I knew it didn't belong inside me, and I wished it would go away. It scared me. It stirred up emotions that made no sense—seething hate, wretched agony, and cold despair—brewing within and directed at myself. This secret I knowingly kept hidden, this Shadow Monster dwelling inside of me, plagued me throughout my school-aged years, and I didn't want anyone to see it. The secret unbeknown to me was that the Shadow Monster stood as the barrier between my conscious mind and the subconscious traumas that remain raw, unhealed, and forgotten.

AM: One of my favorite TV shows growing up in our first house is *Sesame Street,* and I love all of its characters. I can relate firsthand to Cookie Monster's love of chocolate chip cookies, and I sing his "C is For Cookie" song whenever I gobble a cookie myself.

And then there is the lovable monster, Grover. His Super Grover segments and the skits where he plays a waiter are the best. My favorite children's book, *The Monster at the End of This Book,* features Grover.

When I am old enough, I read this book countless times and never tire of it. I remember memorizing it while having it read to me before I can decipher the words. Grover is pictured in the story, pleading with the readers not to turn the page because he heard that there is a monster at the end of the book, and he's afraid to see it. With every page turn, Grover is more and more nervous because he and the readers are getting closer to the finish and closer to the monster he fears. Grover is pictured nailing the book pages shut, bricking them up, pleading with the reader to not finish the book, to just close the book and put it away. But of course, I never put the book down and insist it is read all the way to the end. Spoiler alert: the monster at the end of this book is Grover himself.

Growing up, I have neither insight nor hindsight. I am afraid of the Shadow Monster within me, just as Grover is afraid of the monster at the beginning of his book and all the way through. I know my Shadow Monster is also there in the end, waiting, and I don't want to turn the pages of my life that get me closer to it. Unlike Grover's happy ending, I imagine my Shadow Monster as foreign, an internal enemy, a frightening entity, something other than me. In fact, the Shadow Monster is the protective gatekeeper, guarding all the trauma, sealing it behind closed doors. Unwittingly, by battling against the Shadow Monster, I am fighting against the only shield keeping me safe from the truth, a truth no child is equipped to handle.

As I go forward in my story, I have no more (FM) forgotten memories to share. Every memory I share from this point will be an (AM) always memory. All of the forgotten memories lurk within me beneath the surface, behind the Shadow Monster. I have no way to access them, no way to know they are even there; nevertheless, they manage to haunt my everyday existence.

Section II

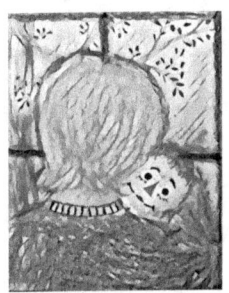

My Normal Family with Abnormal Me

*Mirror, mirror on the wall
that's not really me at all.*

CHAPTER 5

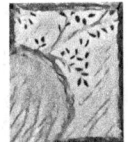

WHAT IS WRONG WITH ME?

No one can figure out why I hyperventilate from time to time, not even me. My hyperventilating episodes start with a tornado drill in fifth grade that scares me into thinking a real tornado is coming, like that scary *The Wizard of Oz* movie where Dorothy and her little dog, Toto, are whisked away to the land with the flying monkeys and the green-faced witch. (Those scenes are too scary to watch on TV, and I hide my face in my hands until they are over.)

Usually, the teacher tells us ahead of time that there is going to be a drill. No such warning occurs today, or if it did, I wasn't paying attention and missed it. As I crouch against the hallway wall in a row with my classmates, all of us in the correct duck and cover position, I brace myself for the tornado to hit us. I begin to gasp, gulping for air as if I can't get enough oxygen to breathe. My teacher notices my fit, but she is unable to calm me. Just then, some firemen appear. The teacher waves them over, and the firemen take me to the nurse's office, where I breathe into a paper bag for the first time. But not the last.

In a few minutes, I recover, and the firemen reassure me that the tornado siren was just a drill. There is no real tornado. I hear that my classmates assume that the firemen were called onto the scene specifically for me, and they think that I went to the hospital. By lunch, the playground rumor has me probably dying. The recess tale is far more impressive than actual events. In fact, the firemen were already in the building ensuring that the safety alarm was ringing properly, and they just happened by as I launched into my breathing frenzy. My mom is called to take me home, and the next day my classmates are relieved to see me back in class, alive.

Even though the tornado drill triggers me into panic mode, I am more disturbed by my long-term female fate. A few days prior to the drill incident, I find out, unbeknownst to me, that my female body will soon bleed every month for about a week. What? I must be the only girl sequestered in the females-only fifth-grade assembly that has no clue about periods. The only period I know about is the punctuation mark at the end of a declarative sentence. Period.

Most of my classmates' moms, including mine, attend this special assembly, fidgeting together in folding chairs toward the back of the gymnasium. I squirm with my friends near the front. The school nurse plays a video explaining menses and covering the bare basics of the birds and the bees. I am appalled. After a brief Q&A, we young ladies are all handed booklet summaries to take home and are dismissed back to class.

Did I give my mom a dirty look as I left the assembly? I sure wanted to but managed a nervous smile instead. I can't quite grasp all of the information I have just heard. I experience shock in my mind, numbness in my body, and anger everywhere. I am mad. Mad I am stuck in this female body. Mad at God for making females bleed. Mad at my mom for not telling me about periods ahead of time—she could have at least told me ahead of the assembly. Mad that boys don't have to go through this bloody morphing. What if I don't ever want to have a baby? All of this bleeding will be just a big waste of time for nothing. No wonder they call it the curse, though the nurse tried to sway us away from using that term. I do feel cursed and inwardly, unspeakably unsettled.

My first hyperventilation incident, which I had hoped was isolated, can be explained. I got scared by the tornado alarm and panicked, end of story. But it didn't end there. I start hyperventilating for no apparent reason, for example, while reading a book in class, or while playing my clarinet in band. This continues at random intervals from fifth-grade school choir to high school cross country. My peers now alert the adult in charge, "She's doing it again," and then dump their lunch contents out, handing me the empty paper bag.

In the foreground of hyperventilating is a background of advancing puberty. My classmates, one girl after another, get their periods, and it is all the buzz amongst the young ladies. Each time, I am relieved it isn't me. In seventh grade, we take a test of 100 questions at the start of the sex education section of Science class. I answer six questions correctly, all I am able to retain from the fifth-grade assembly. The only reason I get an A for the session is because my science teacher grades the sex-ed section strictly on improvement. After the sex-ed instruction is complete, I score 33 out of 100 on the final test.

I can't read about or listen to any of the material, but I don't know why. I always space off instead. To my ears, my teacher sounds like the teachers in the Charlie Brown cartoon specials on TV, "Wah, wah-wah, wah." The words in the textbook blur together incomprehensibly and swirl about on the page. The bell rings, startling me, jerking me back into my seat in time to see the teacher erasing definitions and diagrams from the chalkboard. I shake off my daze, take a deep breath, grab my books, and escape with my classmates, heading down the hall to the next class.

At one point, in junior high, because of my hyperventilation episodes, my parents take me to special doctors for tests. They want to rule out epilepsy or some other seizure disorder. First, I am asked to lie still inside a big tube with flickering lights. I pretend to be gazing at falling stars. It takes a long time. Later, electrodes are glued to my scalp underneath my hair with different colored wires sticking out, all attached to a computer screen with wavy lines and fuzzy images. They ask me to lie down and mimic my hyperventilation breathing. I don't think I can do it on purpose, but they coach me until I do. It feels weird to fake it. Will it yield the same results as the real thing?

I think that I must be dying. Why else would the doctors go to all this fuss? Though the initial idea of death startles me briefly, the reality of this fate doesn't bother me much. So, I won't be around anymore. Big deal. I will just go back to the place where I was before I came here, before I was born, wherever that might be.

A few days later, we got the test results. My parents and I are escorted into a small, private sitting room. I can feel the tension in the air. The doctors report to me and my parents that all of the tests' results are negative. I am crestfallen and brace myself for what difficulties I can expect with this diagnosis. It takes me several thought loops as the adults are talking to realize that negative results are a good thing. To my adolescent brain, negative has always been bad, something you want to avoid. But apparently, in the backward world of medicine, negative means I'm not going to die. I'm not even sick. There is no physical cause for my episodes. They offer a referral to a psychologist. The doctors ask if they should go ahead and schedule the appointment? Mom, Dad, and I search each other's faces for an answer. For all three of us, the answer appears to be a mutual and uneasy no. That won't be necessary.

Glad as I am to not be dying, or even sick, to think that I am instead crazy seems worse, somehow. Maybe it's the Shadow Monster that is making me crazy.

Stuck on a music box
the ballerina spins.
Close the lid again,
trap her in.

Spinning on command is a desperate job,
as is waiting in the dark,
hoping someone lets the light in.
Springing up.

Run, Ballerina, run away!
Unhook your foot,
Flee your prison!
Run, Ballerina, run away,
before they lock you in
to stay.

Chapter 6

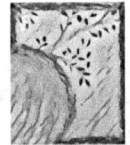

The Heart of a Musician

Mom, she's doing it again," Bigbro tattles on me, shouting for Mom to hear through the swinging kitchen door of our Shady Lane home. He's seven and has just finished practicing his music for his beginning piano lesson.

"Doing what?" Mom calls back, not bothering to come through the door to the piano, where he stands, arms crossed, glaring at me.

I sit my four-year-old self on the piano bench, legs dangling, and plunk back fluently the notes I have just heard my older brother struggle to play. I can't read the music, but I can make the piano keys sound out my brother's songs. It drives Bigbro nuts when I do this without having had any lessons myself. I play "Hot Cross Buns" and "Mary Had A Little Lamb" and whatever new songs he practices.

By the age of five, I get to take piano lessons, too. The piano teacher, Mrs. Carson, lives right across the street from us, so it is easy to get myself to my lessons all by myself and on time. I take to the keyboard right away, using Bigbro's beginner books, and getting through them in no time. I don't recall at what age my brother quits taking piano lessons, but it's a few years later, around the time I am close to catching up to his skill level, and I'll be sharing the same song books. I'm excited that I can read notes now but still rely mostly on my ear. My piano teacher plays all of my new songs for me before sending me home to practice them, so even though I can tell you what the notes are, I don't really have to focus my eyes on the page to play the tunes. By fifth grade, I begin plunking out melodies of my own, composing simple songs similar to whatever lesson skill my music is training me to master.

The dawn of my composing happens to coincide with the first outward appearance of the Shadow Monster—my hyperventilation episodes. My song creation starts as finger doodling, up and down the keyboard until my ear catches a musical phrase it wants to hear again. I connect and rearrange the phrases until a melody appears. I doodle some more to find the accompaniment, and again, it's all a matter of my ear's preference, combining with skills I've mastered. Once a song is born, I practice it repeatedly, over and over, so that the memory of the song is imprinted in my fingers as well as my ears. The tunes are simple at first but pleasant and soothing.

One dazzling afternoon, while the sun's rays dance along my fingers and across the keys, I'm playing and singing a lilting original song when a curious wonder sweeps across my brain. Where's the

Shadow Monster? Is it gone? The hollow at the pit of my stomach where it usually gnaws feels calm, quiet. I pause expectantly. Scan soundlessly. Afraid to disturb the peace. No, not gone, but lulled to sleep. While the Shadow Monster slumbers, my fingers slide across the keyboard, waltzing effortlessly of their own accord, and I breathe in the freedom of the moment. The piano bench secures my temporary break from feeling like a freak, my respite as the rest of the world drifts away, my peace summoned when composing and rehearsing the music in my soul.

In seventh grade, I change piano teachers. My new instructor, Mrs. Snyder, lives in the neighborhood near my junior high school, so one day a week I skip the school bus home and walk to her house. The music is getting advanced enough that I start missing notes—a lot of them. Mrs. Snyder doesn't play any of my lesson pieces for me upon first sight, like Mrs. Carson did. I struggle to read the notes on the page at home on my own, but too many notes are to be played simultaneously and in quick succession. Block chords with four notes in the bass clef knot my fingers and frustrate my ear, wrenching my heart.

    I stop practicing my lesson music and start making up more solos that are fun and tickle my ear, enlivening my heart. When Mom hears me playing the piano at home, she thinks I am practicing my lesson music. Instead, I know I am cheating.

    My piano teacher finally gets fed-up with my abysmal attempts at playing my lesson repertoire and calls my mom. She asks if I've been practicing. My mom answers yes. I sound great at home. Mrs. Snyder arranges for Mom to attend my next lesson. Uh oh!

I'm anxious as I arrive with my mother at my piano teacher's door, tightly clutching my piano books to my chest. As we enter, the two grown-ups exchange pleasantries and again confirm that I am practicing at home every day for at least 30 minutes. Mrs. Snyder pulls up a chair for my mom by the upright piano next to hers. I slump myself on the bench and open the lesson book to my first piece, dreading what I know will be an atrocious performance, at best.

I fix my eyes to the notes on the page, but all my brain sees is a foreign language of ink spots. My fingers strike one key after the other, awkwardly tripping over each other, staggering and landing on one clunker after another, in an endless, obnoxious cacophony of keyboard swears, "Kerplunk, klunk clankety, plunk, clank clunk!" I completely murder the piece of music, and were the composer not already dead, my rendition would surely have killed him.

Mom stares at me, dumbfounded and confused. "That's not the song you've been practicing at home. Play for her what you have been practicing," Mom insists.

Following Mom's command, I set the music aside, take a deep breath, and when I feel my heart calm, begin gliding my fingers across the ivories into a lyrical melody with arpeggio accompaniment. It is an AB form with a bridge, repeating an octave higher and then returning to the original octave. An arc of crescendo and decrescendo sighs within each phrase as the piece resolves in a ritardando. I play my composition flawlessly, as I always do at home.

After the last notes fade, my teacher, breathlessly amazed, says, "I don't know how to teach that!" But she is wise enough not to squelch my potential and skilled enough to also retrain my eyes. From now on, my lessons focus on reading musical notation while playing, and reveling in music all my own, the music that fills my heart and stills the Shadow Monster.

My favorite teacher at Cooper Jr. High School in seventh and eighth grades is, hands down, Mr. Crown. He is as enthusiastic for his love of teaching as he is for the love of his students. Fun spirited, but also no-nonsense, he can crack a corny joke as quickly as he can cast the teacher stink-eye. Both are just to get us squirrely adolescents to pay attention. Of course, he just happens to teach my favorite subjects, as well, music, choir, musical theater, and guitar.

We played ukulele in sixth-grade music class, and I had a blast, so when I saw guitar would be offered in eighth grade, I signed up right away. Mr. Crown has guitars we can use at school, and we can even check one out to practice lessons at home. I quickly adapt to tuning the guitar and to playing the first series of simple chord progressions. For one entire class period, we practiced a strumming style I still use today: down, down-up, up-down-up, in a syncopated 4/4 time. He makes us say it with him as he demonstrates, and we strum along. Down is a quarter note (on beat 1), down-up is two eighth notes (beats 2 &), and up-down-up is three eighth notes (after an eighth rest on the downbeat of 3, strumming on beats & 4 &). This is why I can still effortlessly repeat the saying and the motion in my sleep. Did I mention we practiced the strumming for the entire class period and then reviewed it briefly on other days? Down, down-up, up-down-up. Down, down-up, up-down-up.

Like my study of the piano, I start making up guitar chord progressions with hummed melody lines. In addition to strumming the chords, Mr. Crown teaches us some arpeggio string-plucking patterns. From there, I construct a melancholy lullaby, without words, and, like my original piano songs, it soothes the ever-growing Shadow Monster into submission. I dub it, "The Hummed Lullaby." The title and lyrics to this song don't come right away, not until I've more than doubled my age.

My maternal aunt-by-marriage has a guitar lying around collecting dust and asks do I want it, just to borrow for now, not to have. Of course, I do! Rapt, I strum for hours in my teenage bedroom singing folk songs. Many of my popular piano song books include guitar chord symbols, so I can play current tunes. I also sound out old favorites for which I have no music. And I keep playing my sad original lullaby, which, decades later, becomes "Waiting for Rain."

When our guitar semester is over, Mr. Crown further indulges my composing by letting my friend Mindy and me write a piano song together for a final eighth-grade music project. We create a broken-hearted love ballad for keyboard and voice, like the ones we hear on the radio.

Everyone agrees Mindy is cute. While short for her age, what she lacks in height, she makes up for in spunk. With her brunette locks, whether short or long, she always dons the latest do, from the Dorothy Hamill bob to the wavy styles from *Charlie's Angels*. Her dark hair is a striking contrast to her deep blue eyes. I'm thrilled that she is my friend. We always sit and stand next to each other in chorus for rehearsals and concerts, as we are both sopranos.

In music class, secluded from the rest of our classmates, Mindy and I huddle together in Mr. Crown's small office with an upright piano along an interior window, which overlooks all the comings and goings within the music wing and also the main hall's baby grand. The upright is squished in this corner room among filing cabinets and Mr. Crown's desk with its stacks of music.

The pair of us, Mindy and I, mostly gossip about boys. I end up doing the music songwriting at home to the lyrics we have already made up. Our class session turns into our social time to catch up on who's dating whom: *Did you hear? Did you know? Can you believe it?* Whenever Mr. Crown checks up on us, we can see him coming and immediately launch into song, but are back to our own buzz when he continues on by. In addition to being our final music project, Mr. Crown recommends our song to debut at a local exhibition of musical excellence in the main hall of the art gallery downtown.

Recital exhibition night finally arrives, and Mindy and I are ready. The spacious performance site is the upstairs of the art gallery, with a shiny oak wood floor. White walls surround the hall with individual framed paintings, sparsely hung, and the room, as an art museum, has a high ceiling and good lighting. The middle open space is empty, except for a gorgeous black grand piano and a solo music stand where the instrumentalists will place their sheet music. Two sections of folding chairs line either side of a center aisle, created for the audience to view the space designated as the stage. It reminds me of a wedding venue layout minus the decorations.

The audience, filled with the performers' family members and music teachers, mills about the hall beforehand. Mr. Crown and Mrs. Snyder are there, as are my family and grandparents, and Mindy's family. No one is decked out in formal attire, but instead, dressed in Sunday best. This means knee-length dresses, nylons, and heels for Mindy and me. I'm usually nervous before my piano recitals, but this time, because I am performing my own music, and Mindy is singing, it's more nervous excitement I feel rather than nervous jitters. This is like the adrenaline thrill before dance recitals.

The concert is a distinguished affair of citywide teen talent, all recommended by area music teachers, rather than chosen through audition. I know a few of the other pianists, but most of the budding musicians I haven't seen before tonight. In addition to the pianists, there are a variety of woodwind, brass, and string instrument soloists listed in the program. Mindy and I are the only ones noted performing original music and song lyrics, and Mindy is the only pop singer. Another female vocalist is slated to sing an Italian Art Song.

"Solitude Sunset," our composition, is toward the end of the program, second to last, which is unfortunate for Mindy. As the soloist for our duet, we worry her throat might get dry, and there are a series of high notes in the chorus. She pours a glass of water and carries it to her seat. We position ourselves in chairs opposite each other along the aisle, with our respective families lining the inner seats alongside us.

Once the program begins, the hardest part is sitting still through the ten musicians prior to our turn. The program lists "Solitude Sunset," with music by me, lyrics by both of us, me as accompanist, and Mindy as soprano soloist. As the Cornet Etude performer trumpets his last flourish of notes, Mindy and I lock eyes over her last sip of water. We're up next!

Amidst fading applause, the gentleman emcee steps up front, index cards in hand, and glances at his notes. "Our next duet is a pair of eighth-grade students from Cooper Junior High School, instructed by Mr. Crown. Mindy is a soprano voice student and choir vocalist, and Deborah is an eighth-grade pianist currently taught by Mrs. Snyder. As you can see from your program, Mindy and Deborah are performing an original composition that they wrote together. Let's welcome them to the stage for 'Solitude Sunset.'"

Uplifted by applause, Mindy and I rise in unison and progress to the piano. As we choreographed, she resets the music stand away from the performance area (and the emcee hastily removes it) while I close the heavy piano lid. Posing regally in the crook of the piano, Mindy pauses, waiting as I crank the padded bench seat lower, so my heel can rest on the floor, toes lifted over the sustain pedal. I fold down the music rest and can now clearly see her, and she can peripherally view me.

Mindy looks over her shoulder at me and our eyes lock in silent anticipation... my fingers poised on the keys. Her throat cleared one last time. We share a deep cleansing breath, exhaling our nerves, inhaling our performance aura. Her nod magically launches my fingers into a graceful autopilot, dancing the 4/4 arpeggio introduction before her lilting voice soars—her melody above my baseline, "You just left me standing here and as I watched you walk away, I never thought that I would live to see another sunny day, and as I watched the sunset fade I tried hard not to cry. Now all I have are memories and a pain down deep inside."

The music rises between us, lofting on angel wings, a divine duet—my fingers playing and her voice singing—offering a unison prayer. "The sunset just doesn't seem the same when I'm watching it all alone. I guess I'm just not used to being out here on my own. It just doesn't seem as beautiful when you're not with me here. Soon my sunset... will forever... disappear."

Mindy's vibrato sustains the last note as my arpeggio finale glides up the keyboard, merging with her fermata. We cut off together. Suspending the silence. Momentarily stopping time. Our faces relax, and we exchange deep-cheeked smiles, signaling the applause.

Mindy takes a solo bow. I rise and bow as well, then rush to Mindy's side, grasping her hand for our final joint bow beside the piano. Our hands tingle, surging with the adrenaline of success. As we stare out at our admiring fans, we congratulate ourselves behind ventriloquist-dummy smiles, lips unmoving, speaking for our own ears only. "We did it!" Mindy exclaims.

"I know! Isn't this great?" I agree.

Still floating on the applause, we drop hands and split to rejoin our families in the audience.

A performance afterglow enlivens the hall. With Mr. Crown and Mrs. Snyder, Mindy and I join the other musicians and their teachers in a receiving line running the length of one wall. We're congratulated by strangers and family alike, with praises and accolades that dizzy my brain and lift my spirits. I'm both self-conscious from their compliments and proud of our accomplishments, my cheeks dimpling with a permanent flush.

As the receiving line disperses, my dad calls me over to introduce me to a man I don't recognize. I notice they have been chatting with each other at the hall entrance for some time.

"Deborah, someone would like to meet you," my dad motions me to stand alongside the two of them, "this is my fourteen-year-old daughter, Deborah."

The man, smartly dressed and almost handsome, looks gray around the edges of his dark sideburns. He reaches out to shake my hand. "Let me introduce myself," he hands me his business card with one hand and firmly grasps the other. I return the solid handshake. This new acquaintance repeats to me what it says on the card, his name, and his title as a talent agent for an entertainment company with an address in California. "You see, I think you have that special something we look for in the music industry. You could be the next Olivia Newton John!"

Dad pipes in, "I told him you sing, too."

I'm as taken aback as I am flattered. My dad and this man talk in front of me about my Dad's brother in California. It could likely be arranged for me to live with his brother and his family in San Diego. I am hesitant and half-dumbfounded at the possibilities they are discussing about the route to potentially becoming a teenage popstar. The thought of stardom dizzies me, and the conversation ends with the agent telling us to stay in touch, requesting that we let him know what we decide. "It is so nice to meet you, Deborah. I hope to be working with you soon in sunny California."

A few long-distance phone calls later between my dad and his brother, and, yes, I can live with my uncle in California if I want to pursue a music career. Fortunately, the decision is up to me, and whatever I want to do is fine. If I choose to go to California, I will get to live with my favorite cousin, Justine, at her house.

Justine is my age, minus two months, to the day. Her brother, my other cousin, is just two days older than Bigbro. The summer Justine and I are aged five, right before we both start kindergarten, my family takes a long camping trip in the family station wagon to visit her and her family. I am amazed at how close she lives to a real zoo, and better yet, to Disneyland! We even go to the ocean, but I am afraid of getting bitten by the crabs that I imagine are everywhere hiding in the seaweed wads washed up on the beach. It's hard not to be jealous of Justine. Not only does she live in California, but she is pretty and smart. She can already read, and her parents have money to spare, so she seems to get whatever she wants, including a four-poster bed with a lacy canopy.

As soon as we are old enough to write, Justine and I become long-distance pen-pals, and I anxiously await her weekly letters. My very first piano composition I write is for her, and I name it after her. When we are twelve, just after sixth grade and before starting junior high, my uncle makes me a gracious offer to fly me to California on my own for a visit with Justine.

My first time on a plane is thrilling. I'm not afraid to travel alone. In fact, I prefer it to the forced hours of an endless boring car ride trapped with my family. When it's just me, I breathe easy. A nice lady attendant looks out for me, making sure I make it all the way to my destination, since I am flying alone. Ever since this first airplane ride, every time I take off, and I feel the surge of the engines thrusting me airborne, I think, "What a miracle it is to be flying in the sky!" and marvel at this metaphysical experience.

My twelve-year-old self looks down through the tiny window and sees a patchwork quilt of squares, country roads outlining the farm fields below, and the wandering intersections of woods and rivers interrupting the otherwise perfect pattern. The little cars look like ants crawling about until the landscape disappears altogether. Flying in the sky feels safer than being on the ground. Rising further, we break through the cloud cover and now only clouds as far as my eye can see, white fluffy ones that shape themselves into stuffed animals. I see a fuzzy rabbit, then a cuddly bear and a cute whale—friendly critters billow everywhere.

Once in San Diego, Justine's house has an in-ground backyard pool shaped like a kidney bean. We spend most of our time in our two-piece swimsuits, reeking of cocoa butter, tanning next to the pool on lounge chairs, like Hollywood glamour girls, listening to pop music on a transistor radio. On a solitary rainy day, we nest on the living room floor by the stereo and call in to a local radio station to request our favorite songs all afternoon long. We shriek with delight when they announce the ones we've picked, and we sing and dance along.

Twelve is old enough to wander around Disneyland on our own, which takes up a whole day. The same is true for SeaWorld, where I've never been, and I purchase a Shamu the Whale stuffed animal souvenir to take home. Our day at the beach is cold and windy, too chilly for swimming in the ocean, but overall it is a delightful trip.

But now, contemplating my musical prospects from age fourteen, the thought of going back to San Diego to live is enticing. But do I really want to go?

The Shadow Monster, who's grown from an uneasy nuisance into an obnoxious hindrance, constantly gnaws away at my self-esteem, leaving me off-kilter and frail. It grumbles in my subconscious loud enough to be almost heard and rumbles my stomach with a big no. I'm thrillingly tempted, but my girlfriends and I have flipped through too many tragedies in the teenage tabloid rags about alcohol abuse, drug overdoses, and suicide among the young, rich, and famous. Do I really want to move all the way to California right before my freshman year of high school? Am I willing to leave Mindy, Lenee, and Jodie behind? What about Great-Grandma? What about my horse, Dawn? Do I really think I'm good enough to be a teen music idol? It seems like a lot of pressure with no guarantees. Shadow Monster or not, I decide it's not for me. Am I too scared? Yes. Is it for good reason? Yes. Do I understand why? Not completely. But the overarching vision that comes to me in my mind's eye is me dying in my early twenties from mismanaged stardom.

I lurk as the Loch Ness Monster,
rarely emerging for air,
the art of holding my breath, mastered, but unnatural.
Living beneath the surface,
struggling to remain still in a tornado undertow,
not wanting to pop open the splashguard to the sky.
No gills sustain me
during shifting tides between tidal waves.

Chapter 7

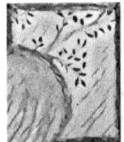

Coming of Age

Finally, it's my turn. The summer I am aged 14, just after finishing the eighth grade, I get my first period while riding in the family station wagon on vacation, en route to the Lake of the Ozarks. I find out in a gas station restroom and flag down my mom in hushed tones to tell her I've sprung a leak. Lilbro sees I need a change of underwear from my suitcase and starts laughing and singing the classic kid "Diarrhea" song, "some people think it's funny, but it's really dark and runny, diarrhea, diarrhea…," complete with underarm fart-noise interjections. Bigbro tells him that's not what's going on with me, but he can't get Lilbro to pipe down. Undeterred, Lilbro continues to taunt me with a classic younger-brother point, laughing at me that I pooped my pants.

It's easy to ignore Lilbro's annoying antics because he genuinely has no clue about girls and periods. What's hard to bear is riding in the car with the rest of my family, who are fully aware that I'm menstruating. Why couldn't this have happened at home so I could hide in my room until it was over? Instead, I slump in the back seat, squished next to my brothers, avoiding eye contact, fighting back stinging tears, wishing I could disappear, and feeling conspicuous and humiliated. Leaning my head against the window, I stare at the scenery blurring by, feeling the Shadow Monster lumbering within me. My mind is numbing out again, unable to discern the family conversation, spacing off, drifting away.

Suddenly the car—lurching onto crunching gravel—jars me back into my body. Hours must have passed. We are pulling up to the lakeside cabin, our home for the next week.

After this holiday, I begin ninth grade at Hillside High School. In the middle of the fall semester of ninth grade, though I have had my share of short-term boyfriends since the sixth grade, I meet my first love—my high school sweetheart, Jack. He's slightly taller than the average-sized me, has dark hair, blue eyes, and a quick smile. He is smart, cute, and funny and, best of all, he loves me. We are in marching band and concert band together—he's in the saxophone section, and I'm with the clarinets. I also join the cross-country team, not because I love running, but because it is the only coed sports team at school and Jack loves running—he's good at it. If I want to see him at all during cross-country season, I had better sign up, too. My only goal for cross-country is to never finish a race in last place. I achieve this goal but rarely finish the season with my teammates, quitting once it gets too cold and the season is almost over anyway. I only letter in the sport one year.

As with many first loves, Jack and I give each other our virginity—at least, that's how my mind sees it—and even if I could have recalled my abuse history, which I can't, this is my first consensual sexual encounter. We are both aged 15, in his upstairs bedroom, shy and eager in our new nakedness with each other. From what I have been taught in sex-ed, penetration might hurt a bit at first for the woman. It did, but not enough for me to stop it. Jack seems to really enjoy himself. When we finish our first time, though I am pleased with this milestone moment, I think, that's it? I don't get what all the fuss is about. I didn't really feel anything but numb and frozen. Even so, it becomes the norm for the pair of us to have sex whenever we find a chance time alone together. I play along for his sake, and because the act is considered risqué for teenagers, but I never get much out of it. I can feel his weight, his thrusting, his erotic breathing, but otherwise nothing. I stare at the ceiling and wait. I much prefer just kissing and making out together. I never orgasm. Not during sex. Not on my own. I don't even know what an orgasm is or that it is possible for me to have one. That pleasant surprise comes years later.

Though the school frowns on public displays of affection in the hallways (PDAs as they are nicknamed), Jack and I often hold hands on the way to our respective classes and make out at our lockers. We go to Band class together and occasionally other class subjects. It happens that we are in the same ninth-grade English class with Mrs. Grey.

Mrs. Grey knows my maternal grandmother and is around her age. I find her strict, running her classroom as if she has had military training, expecting rapt attention and silence from her students. I tire from being on my best, soldier-like behavior for the entire 50 minutes of her class period. Still, I like English as a subject, even if Mrs. Grey isn't my favorite teacher.

In the previous three quarters, I earn all A's. I love writing. I would rather write an essay than take an exam any day. So far, we did nonfiction essay writing and reporting, creative-fiction writing, and then poetry reading and writing. This final quarter is English literature. Reading isn't my favorite thing to do, especially when someone else picks out the books. But I manage to make it through Shakespeare's flowery language in *Romeo and Juliet* and do okay on the comprehension test. But then trouble comes with Charles Dickens's *Great Expectations*.

I do not like to read because it activates the creative thinking part of my brain where the Shadow Monster can seep through. When I read something scary or creepy, my emotions trigger and begin to bubble within me, trying to surface. Something about actively engaging fictional characters in an inner fantasy world of danger and distress threatens my wellbeing. *Great Expectations* is one of those scary books. Why is it required reading?

So, in English class, the fifteen-year-old me cracks open the famous novel. The first scene with Pip meeting the convict on the moors creeps me out a bit, but it is Miss Havisham and Estella that I can't stomach.

Miss Havisham remains her own captor. She traps herself in her house because of past trauma—she was abandoned by the love of her life on her wedding day. I find her character and the environment she chooses to inhabit beyond sickening until I can't continue turning the pages. Her manipulation of the cold Estella makes everything worse.

I freeze at my desk, numb, staring at the page, unable to read a single word. Day after day in that English class, I am in an almost trancelike state, making no sense of anything on the pages. There is a girl within me, who I can't reach, who is stirred by the novel's fantasy world, and she is just like Miss Havisham.

I can feel this deranged, tortured soul, this… me, stirring beneath the surface, but she is nowhere tangible to be found. My search to find where she lurks within me is as murky as the moors in the story. I feel as demented as Miss Havisham for identifying so strongly with her, as if I am her. Additionally, part of me is as stoic and emotionally numb as Estella. It is nearly impossible to bear my inner haunting. I don't know how I manage to stay in my seat, day after day, hour after hour, minute after minute, instead of running, screaming from that classroom.

Even though Jack helps me study for the final comprehension test with *Cliff Notes*, Mrs. Grey is too smart to use any of these questions on her test. It is multiple choice and I still fail miserably, turning out to be a below-average guesser. My teacher does consult with me on why I didn't read the book. Do I tell her about the Shadow Monster? No. Do I tell her about Mrs. Havisham and Estella and me being some sort of morphed hybrid psychopath? No. Mrs. Grey dislikes my fake explanation. I didn't know what else to say to her other than I found the story boring and the characters uninteresting.

Just as we did after completing *Romeo and Juliet*, our class reward for concluding the *Great Expectations* portion of the curriculum is we get to watch the full-length movie version of the book over the next week of class sessions. It's the black and white 1946 rendition, and it reminds me of what a horror movie would be, if I had ever seen one. I hide my head in my hands, trying not to look, just like when I watch the scary parts of *The Wizard of Oz*. (In a twisted coincidence, I was a Lollipop Guild member of Munchkinland in the year's high school musical.) Which is worse: reading *Great Expectations* in print and letting my imagination fill in the blanks, or seeing it acted out on the screen in front of me? I squirm in my desk and cry silently. Even though the room is dark, and no one can see me, I need to leave—now. I raise my hand, signaling Mrs. Grey. She crouches by my desk to avoid casting her shadow across the screen. "I don't feel well," I whisper, "I need to go to the nurse's office."

"Okay, you may be excused," she whispers permission, never expecting a student to feign illness on a movie day.

The bright lights from the hallway blast my eyes. I breathe a heavy sigh, relieved to be free from that classroom. With each step I take toward the nurse's office, my headache intensifies, from a nagging pulse to a pounding migraine.

Neither my first migraine nor my last, the resulting phone call to my mom releases me from school to recuperate at home for a couple of days. The intense headaches seem to correlate with my menstrual cycle, making my head hurt slightly more than my awful cramps. The Curse is the proper name for my periods, regardless of what the elementary school nurse said all those years ago. And, for whatever reason, my monthlies are not at regular intervals but spring up after three weeks, or after six, and last randomly long, with heavy flow the whole time. I hate them. Even when I am well enough to go to school, I cannot concentrate. Their unpredictable nature mirrors my God-awful mood swings. My experience seems out of proportion to that of my girlfriends. Everyone else takes Pamprin and still attends PE class. Not me. I am down and out, unfit for public interaction. Sometimes, like today, when I was excused from watching that awful Dickens movie, the migraines just come on their own, regardless of whether or not I'm flowing. My mom also gets migraines. It must be hereditary.

The ominous Shadow Monster lurks ever closer to the surface each passing month as my sadness looms, beyond measure, beyond explanation, beyond hiding, until I can no longer pretend that I am a happy-go-lucky teenager. By junior year, my depression can't be quelled, though no apparent reason exists for me to be depressed: I have a good family, I have a steady boyfriend, I get decent grades (except that weird F for the last quarter of Freshman English class), I have friends from my band and choir activities, and I attend all the sporting events and dances. Outside of school, I have a part-time cashier job, I ride my horse and play the piano. I am an average, middle class, teenage kid. Nevertheless, one school day, while meeting Jack for lunch in a secluded corner of the outdoor atrium, I burst into tears and confess I want to die, but I don't know why.

"I just feel awful all the time," I sob, "I think I hate myself. Why would I hate myself?"

"You don't hate yourself, you're just having a bad day," he consoles me, wrapping his arm around my shoulders, sheltering me from onlookers.

"You don't understand, it's not just a bad day, it's every day. I just never told you because I didn't want you to break up with me for being a depressed weirdo."

"I'm not breaking up with you," he reassures me and adds, "and I've always been a bigger weirdo than you."

I smile through my tears but continue, "I'm serious, Jack. I can't live like this anymore."

He expels a heavy breath, "Well, then we better get you some help. Maybe you should talk to the school counselor after lunch and tell him what you just told me."

I resist his plan, but he persuades me that it will be okay, that it doesn't matter what other people think, that going to a counselor isn't a bad thing.

After lunch, I reluctantly report to the counselor's office and burst into tears all over again. I don't want him to tell my parents, but he claims he must, so he does. He hands me a note excusing me from class for the rest of the day, and gives me an appointment card scheduling me to meet with the district psychiatrist, where I get my first antidepressant prescription.

I officially label myself crazy. It's no longer a private matter between me, myself, and I. I cannot hide from my peers that I am dismissed from class to attend my on-site therapy sessions or am excused to the nurse's office to take my medication. Perhaps those doctors trying to diagnose my hyperventilation episodes in junior high were right: it's all in my head and I need a shrink. In the early '80s, receiving mental health services is taboo. Why are my brain chemicals messed up? Just a fluke of nature, I guess. All I know is that I am internally, incredibly unstable, and sad, despite my happy exterior role-playing. I feel like a fraud and a fake. It takes a lot of effort to be me. I carry the internal weight of self-loathing that I attribute to the Shadow Monster and try my best to ignore the gloom so that I can act the part of a functioning teenager. The Shadow Monster is winning, but I still don't mention the Shadow Monster's existence to anyone.

*Here she comes now,
there she goes,
where she'll stop
nobody knows,
swirling in the sands of time
without reason,
without rhyme,
chasing after shooting stars,
never mind how far they are,
always hoping that she'll find
the intermingling of
all-souls divine.*

Chapter 8

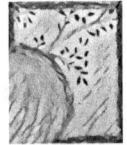

Cinnamon & Dawn

The summer I'm age seven, the summer of forgetting, is the summer my family moves from Shady Lane to the small acreage on Fossil Ridge Road. The newer olive-green ranch house nestles down a hillside that slopes away from the road, with a walkout basement and sliding glass door on its west end. The grass surround is dotted with evergreens and apple trees, while maples line the roadway. To the north, the lawn opens to a lean-to style barn and a couple of grassy pastures, fenced in by barbed wire.

Stretching the length of our property to the west is a deep, wooded ravine with a narrow creek snaking through the bottom. My brothers and I invite friends, and our kid-sized sneakers tromp down steep banked footpaths that crisscross the ravine floor, leading us to the stream. In summers, the sinewy waterway is home to slippery frogs, silvery minnows, and painted turtles that we catch and release. Tracking hoof and paw prints beneath our own treads, we discover rabbit burrows, deer grass beds, squirrel nests, raccoon tree hollows, and beaver dams. The fox and coyotes howl at night, but it is hard to discern their imprints from those left by roaming country dogs. In winters, we dam up the creek, forcing the water out of its banks to cover the ravine floor in a wilderness rink of ice. Padded beneath layers of down coats, wool scarves, and knit hats, we remove our mittens long enough to lace up our skates for an afternoon of gliding around our woodland ice arena.

Our family's collection of pets expands with the open spaces we inhabit in the country. Soon after moving, we take in a stray dog, Tramp. He has the color markings of a collie, with the build and short fur of a German shepherd. The poor thing's ribs are prominent, and he's skittish, especially around men. I coax him with treats until he lets me pet him, then cuddle him—my reward: an abundance of face licks and loyalty. His silent company, his deep listening, his soulful gaze comfort me when I first sense the Shadow Monster's presence. Tramp knows when I'm sad, sits with me while I cry, and licks away my tears until I'm ready to wrestle and play with him again.

Another stray comes along—Smokey—a tiny, tortoiseshell kitten that my brothers find by the roadside. I help nurse her with an eyedropper until she can drink from a bowl. The cat, who my parents insist will live outside in the barn once she's grown, sits on my lap while I sit on the couch watching TV, purring away the angst of my day. Smokey's purrs smooth my emotional turbulence, and she soothes my aching heart with her unconditional love, then her playful antics revive my spirit as she bats and chases a ball I roll across the floor.

An empty barn and pasture are not complete without horses. Cinnamon, a pony for us kids, comes first. Her brown fur is the color of cinnamon (thus her name), with a black mane and tail and eyes almost as dark. She loves being brushed with a currycomb, which I am happy to indulge, smoothing her soft coat to a silky sheen. Cinnamon is soon followed by my mom's appaloosa, Cheetah.

As the proud owner of a pony, I join 4-H. Cinnamon and I win a red ribbon for Halter Showmanship at the county fair and a blue for Western Saddle riding. I find this ironic, as the ease of training for each of these events is the other way around. She is a gentle lead but a stubborn mount. We have a battle of wills with every ride. At the local rodeo, we do well with the Pony Express obstacle course, not placing, but improving our middle-of-the-pack timing. I look forward to making a good showing in my last competition for the evening—barrel racing. I have practiced hours with Cinnamon, galloping around the three-barrel triangular weave pattern, and hope to improve our time enough to place for a ribbon.

The crowd is stacked up in the bleacher-lined arena, decked out in straw cowboy hats and giant belt buckles, leather cowgirl boots and ponytail ribbons. The base scent of saddle soap, horse sweat, and road apples swirls in the breeze, mingling with freshly munched popcorn. As the dust settles from the last racer, my azure Western shirt's pearl snaps reflect the arena floodlights. With a tip of my white hat, I signal the starting flagger

that I'm ready, and the loudspeaker tenor voice announces, "Next up in the Junior Pony Class is Deborah riding Cinnamon.
"She's ready to race.
"Five. Four. Three. Two. One."
The flag drops. I kick Cinnamon with my heels, "Yah! Yah! Yah!" bracing for her lunge off the starting line. But nothing: no surge of force beneath me, no thunder of hooves kicking up dust, no sprint to seize the pattern, no competitive spirit. Instead, Cinnamon trots, jogging around the first barrel, her short-stride steps clop, clop, clopping, ignoring my heel kicks, rein waves, and yips urging her to go faster. The amplified voice says, "Oh no! That's not what you want to see...." My frenzied effort is in vain for all to witness as she continues her defiant trot around barrel number two. "Maybe she can get a little gallop out of her yet...." Barrel number three, and she is still obstinately trotting, and I give up playing the flailing fool, just praying for this longest ride of my life to end. "Nope. Oh well, maybe next time. Let's give her a nice round of applause for finishing anyway! Deborah and Cinnamon from the 4-H Club, Sunset Saddlers!" The crowd applauds politely as we finish dead last beneath the spotlights.

I am convinced that Cinnamon lost on purpose, being her stubborn self, just to show me who's boss. I could blame the venue and her being nervous, had we not already successfully completed the Pony Express race. That is Cinnamon for you! Her stubborn streak tutors me in the stamina of determination, the tenacity of staying power, and the value of finishing what I've started—even when things do not go as planned.

The rodeo fiasco is not why we sell Cinnamon. My 11-year-old legs are outgrowing her pony size, and my brothers rarely ride anymore. Some family friends of ours have a horse for sale that is green-broke (meaning she has just learned to accept a rider on her back) that I've already ridden and love. Her name is Dawn.

Dawn is ours the summer before I start sixth grade. She is an average quarter horse, sorrel colored, with a mane and tail to match. A white star in the middle of her forehead stripes down the length of her nose. Her spirit is sweet, gentle, easy-going. I can let go of the struggle that came with our stubborn pony and just enjoy Dawn's soft, swift stride.

My friends and I revel in cowgirl adventures at my house, if it's nice enough for horseback riding. With Cinnamon, we cowgirls were limited to riding together two at a time on her back, with me at the reins, the experienced handler, galloping within our fenced pastures in case she was in one of her willful moods. Now that we have Dawn, I usually ride Cheetah and let my guests ride the gentle Dawn, and we can ride up to four at a time, two on each horse instead of taking turns. While riding Dawn and Cheetah, my friends and I know the freedom of leaving the perimeter of our fenced property and galloping the back roads.

Though riding with friends amuses me, I cherish riding on my own. Solo rides with Dawn, like composing my own songs, soothe the Shadow Monster: my piano playing sings the lullaby; my horseback riding rocks the cradle. Even when brushing her, I'm free.

Dawn becomes my sole companion. From cherishing my girlish secrets to cradling my adolescent growth spurts, from serving as a vessel for my teenage heartbreaks and then offering her neighs of compassion and whinnies of approval, her sighs of understanding and murmurs of blessing, she is a friend like no other.

Dawn is as eager as I to escape the confines of her pastures and go for a ride, her ribs bellowing between my thighs. Her gait flows from easy steps to rhythmic trots, from shuffling hooves to steady loping glides. I breathe as one with her breath, one with her stride, one with her power—two beasts, her and me, morphing into a mythical creature. I think if I ride long enough, far enough, fast enough, I will outrun this world—or at least leave it for a time. My blonde locks and her sorrel shock canter in the breeze. As empty sky and rushing grass meet our steady core, we are one in the same. Here is peace, my temple body, my Zen mind, my transparent soul.

Something beyond this world is holy, and Dawn whisks me there, lilting in the liminal, swirling in the sacred, and dangling in the divine. Here I find my own north star, the enduring me, the eternal me, the emblazoned me that still shines from before my birth, within my current life, and beyond what my lifetime is able to hold. Dawn is an oracle, offering me a prayer, a canticle, a communion, an ascension, all in a day's ride.

*But there were birthday cakes
and holidays
and Disney on TV,
games to play
pictures to take
vacation times
and nursery rhymes,
and all the spaces in between
with family and friends.
This is all a part of who I am.*

CHAPTER 9

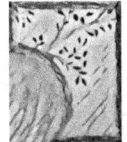

ON A GIVEN SUNDAY

My parents, high school sweethearts in the late 1950s, got married soon after my Mom graduated from high school, as my dad had graduated the year prior. They exchanged traditional marriage vows at the altar of my mom's family's Lutheran church, and before long, my dad joins this LCA denomination.

I am baptized here and confirmed here. Because of this church community, I attend summer Bible camp away from home for a week, several summers in a row. With my Sunday school classmates, I compete in girls' basketball and softball leagues, and I join the youth group for lock-ins (teen overnights in church basements), mingling with kids from local LCA churches. Here are my first musical opportunities, singing with the children's choir and the youth choir, ringing handbells, and piping with the recorder ensemble, all of which blend as part of the worship services. Much of my young life revolves around this congregation and the generations of my mother's side of the family who attend with us.

Just as Sunday mornings are for church, and Sunday afternoons are for Mom's scrumptious pot roast dinners, Sunday evenings are for devouring fistfuls of popcorn and watching the *Wonderful World of Disney* on TV, "in living color." Dad makes the best popcorn, using an aluminum pan with a flat lid on the stove. To keep the kernels from burning, he shakes the pan. As the popcorn starts to lift the lid, he dumps part of the white fluff into the large, yellow Pyrex bowl and returns to shaking the pan until the corn is all popped to perfection. Then Dad melts the butter and drizzles it ever so evenly across the top layer of popcorn. That's when the magic begins. With a quick flick of his wrists, the popcorn arcs up above the bowl and lands back within, shifting the top kernels to the bottom and the bottom kernels to the top. More butter drizzling. More tossing of popcorn. He can get it to fly amazingly high before catching it on the rebound, rarely missing a single piece.

When I am not watching Dad in the kitchen, my brothers and I lie on the floor in front of the TV, resting our elbows to hold our heads in our hands. *Mutual of Omaha's Wild Kingdom* is on while Dad pops our supper snack. We are fascinated by all of the animals and also amused that Jim does all the fieldwork while Marlin Perkins simply narrates from a safe distance away. Between the animal scenes and the Mutual of Omaha commercials, the popcorn bowl is heaping, and we eagerly claim our seats on the couch to watch the opening cartoon fireworks around Cinderella's Palace and just in time for Tinker Bell to wave her magic wand and begin the show.

My favorite memories from our Sunday traditions are being in church, sandwiched between my grandma and my great-grandma in our red-cushioned pew. Our pew is rows back on the right side, facing the altar and nearest the center aisle. Because Mom and Dad are in the choir lofts up front, on either side of the altar, wearing their long flowing robes, my wriggly brothers and I need our grandmas' supervision during the service. The organ prelude booms melodic, with brilliant fanfare coursing through the pipes as we wait for the service to begin. When I am my smallest, I scribble pictures on the attendance cards with the golf-scoring-sized pencils, proudly showing both grandmas my art.

As I grow, I love singing the melody to the hymns while standing between Grandma's alto part in my left ear and Great-Grandma's monotone in my right ear. Hymns in stereo. I'm not sure if Great-Grandma's off-key renditions are due to her hearing loss or if she's always been tone-deaf. Either way, it does not prevent her from belting out the words to her own tune. We are a discordant trio made in heaven.

At offering time, my elders hand my brothers and me their sealed envelopes to place into the shiny gold plate as it passes by and then provide a mint or stick of gum to occupy us during the never-ending sermon. I painstakingly unwrap the candy in slow motion, preventing the crackling paper from disrupting the hush of the sanctuary, and then alternately curl up in one elder's lap and then the other's, as my mouth, full of flavor and rhythmic motion, along with their comforting embraces, relieve the boredom.

The best Sundays are when we have Sunday dinner out together after church at the American-style buffet. Church just isn't church anymore after my grandmothers pass away in my mid-teens—first Great-Grandma, soon followed by Grandma, dying just six months later. There are holes left in our hearts, penned lines in our family tree, and vacant cushions in the pews where my maternal matriarchs used to be.

Growing up, I have my own inner sense of God that often contradicts what the adults teaching Sunday School and Confirmation have to say about him. I'm all about the questions, trying to get the instructors to see the flaws in their religious logic.

"You have to believe in Jesus and accept him as your Savior to go to Heaven," says one very certain old lady teacher.

"What about my Jewish friends? They don't get to go to heaven?"

"No."

"What about tribes in Africa who have never had a chance to be taught about Jesus? They don't get to go to heaven even though they have no way of knowing who he is?"

"Well… um… a… no. All I know is that you have to accept Jesus as your savior or you can't get into heaven… so I guess not." Her certainty wains as if she has never considered such an obvious scenario before now.

I don't agree with her or anyone who tells me Jesus is the only way to get to heaven. "Jesus loves me this I know," is the song I love to sing. And if Jesus loves me, he loves everyone, all of us, just the same. I maintain that in heaven, it's either all of us or none of us. I don't believe in hell, except that I've decided, if there is a hell, it is on earth, for the simple reason that Adam and Eve were kicked out of the Garden of Eden paradise and then punished by being left to roam the earth. They weren't sent somewhere else for punishment, to some other hell, but earth was their punishment location. These young beliefs carry me along from elementary through high school.

In my early teen years, Great-Grandma is too frail to attend church, and Dad declares himself an atheist. Every Sunday morning, from then on, I lie in bed and anticipate the godless disruption of my parents arguing about whether or not we are going to church as a family. Ever since my dad declared he doesn't believe in that stuff anymore, he refuses to be a hypocrite and go to church. It was never a question before—it is what we do—go to church together, every single Sunday, with a rare exception granted due to illness. Embracing my teenage self, I am content to sleep in and stay home, but the angst of their verbal impasse ties knots in my stomach. Our new routine is Mom crying every Sunday morning and then either attending church with a begrudging husband and family in tow or with only one to three kids going with her, a gesture we kids make because of the guilt we feel over her hurt feelings. I am usually one of the kids to go to church with her, but once in a while, I stay home. Just because. Whether I decide to stay or go, I never feel good about my choice, knowing that, either way, my mom is feeling emotionally defeated and terribly alone. This goes on for months. I now hate Sundays.

HAZEL'S LAMP

Spotlight,
    center stage.
With spirit
        I fly,
casting shadows of my own—
just one.

I am one
    with the light,
        song of my own
        being, making the stage
                        fly
                With my spirit.

The audience has spirit
    that is one
with me; they fly
    into the light
    to share my stage,
    yet each on their own.

"No one can own
    Your spirit,"
Hazel said, "Your stage
is the one
    to light
        your way, so fly!
"Fly,
    on your own
        toward the light
    so your spirit
        can be one
            with you — off stage."

Hazel reached that stage
    where she needed to fly.
I was the only one
    she told of coming to her own,
    of how her spirit
        danced in the light.

Now, I'm on my own
    and seek her spirit,
            her light.

Chapter 10

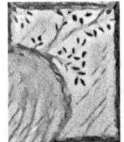

My Twin Soul

My maternal great-grandma and I have a special bond from the time I am an infant, or so I'm told. As a baby, Mom claims Great-Grandma always smoothed out my blankets. She couldn't have me lying on a wrinkle. That would not do. To this day, I detest sleeping on wrinkles in my sheets, a kind of *Princess and the Pea* problem I must have learned from her fussing over me. I just know that while I am growing up, whatever my age, wherever Great-Grandma is, that's where I want to be. Her presence is magical to me.

She looks elderly thin, with laugh lines adorning her twinkling, hazel eyes and creased cheeks revealing a lips-only smile. Her gray tuft of hair is set by "her gal" at the beauty parlor once a week, keeping her locks waved into a short bun at her nape. Like a deer, Great-Grandma's exterior presentation is elegant, quiet, and still, as she blends into the scenery without notice. But I notice her and feel her inner wonderment, alive and overflowing.

I think of us as twin souls. Great-Grandma and I are nearly conjoined at every family gathering, observing the rest of the family and then laughing at our own inside jokes, never spoken aloud. We don't read each other's minds, we experience the world through the same lens and happen to think the exact same things at the exact same time. Extended family members are aware of our cahoots-like behavior, which they deem odd, and comment on it. "What are those two always laughing at?" is a commonly overheard inquiry, which makes us laugh even harder. We are both thinking, "You! We're laughing at you," without saying so. The pair of us find our extended family members ridiculously funny and a source of endless amusement. Watching them is like watching a beloved sitcom. (I guess that makes us the canned laughter?)

Twin souls, two generations removed, with identical thoughts—this is Great-Grandma and me. I am too young to question this or to know how rare our joint perception is. It doesn't even occur to me that she is the only person I relate to in this mystical way.

Great-Grandma moved to live with her daughter's (my grandma's) family at some point after becoming a widow. My mom must have been around high school age when the move-in happened, as I've seen pictures of my teenage-looking mother and my great-grandma's dog (Buttons) as a puppy. I was privileged to briefly know and love Buttons. By the time I came along, it was just Grandma and Great-Grandma and Buttons living in the house my mom grew up in—a white, two-story house set back from a bustling, two-lane, city street.

Barometric pressure changes activate terrible bouts of arthritis in Great-Grandma's joints, especially in her long, weathered fingers and her often swollen knees. She lies on the davenport in the dining room with the shades drawn, a bottle of Bufferin and a glass of water on the end table. "I wouldn't wish this on my worst enemy," I recall her saying on more than one occasion. Grandma orders that we kids play quiet as church mice so as not to disturb Great-Grandma's convalescence.

When she is feeling well, Great-Grandma and I take slow walks around the block, pausing often. We see jagged lines of red ants crawling between the cracks of the sidewalk and wonder silently together (in our parallel thinking) where they are going. Our attention turns to a robin perched on a sloped branch of a cherry tree, "Let's wait to see if she sings to us before she flies away," we mutually think. We watch. Sometimes the robin bursts into a flurry of chirps, singing to us, her rapt audience, as we, in our heads, cheer and applaud her marvelous song; or sometimes, the robin silently flits away, and we think, "Maybe she'll sing to us another day." We share these encounters without uttering a sound, exchanging glances of an easy peace together, blessed moments of harmonious quietude. This silence, filled with our combined knowing, is sacred, and I take it for granted, even though I sadly realize Great-Grandma won't live forever.

I pick flowers as we turn toward home, collecting yellow dandelions and purple violets from the grassy parking strip in a bouquet to give to Grandma back at the house. Grandma puts them in Dixie cups of water on the kitchen windowsill, even as she declares,

"These aren't flowers, they're weeds." I can tell she is touched by my gesture, even as she pretends to criticize because she can't quite hide the one upturned lip corner of a smile.

On days not nice enough for strolling, Great-Grandma and I sit and color at the kitchen table with or without my siblings and other cousins. I love my grandma's kitchen table. It is a corner booth with a bench seat along the back wall, and looks like a '50s style eatery. Regular kitchen chairs line the open sides. This is where all the coloring happens. Crayons, coloring books, and the blank-sided sheets of inventory papers from the grocery store, where my grandma works as a cashier, spread out around us. Great-Grandma and I draw and color at one end of the table while, at the other end, Grandma reads *Reader's Digest*, chain-smoking cigarettes and drinking bottomless cups of steaming black coffee. Grandma loves to interject with jokes and puns from her magazine and then stifles audible giggles of her amusement. Great-Grandma and I either groan or laugh along with her, depending on the humor, but invariably have a joint response.

My grandmothers don't have a car between them since neither of them drive. My grandma either walks or takes the bus to work. She does weekly grocery shopping one evening a week, and my mom's siblings' families rotate on who drives to the store since she cannot carry home a week's worth of groceries by herself after her cashier shifts. I love the days when it's our family's turn to take her to the store. Everyone at the grocer's knows my grandma and stops to talk to us.

And Grandma always rewards us with a dozen-and-a-half frosted cake donuts from the store's onsite donut machine to take home for our family to share. There are always six with white frosting, six with caramel frosting, and six with chocolate frosting, some with and some without nut sprinkles. Best donuts ever!

One Saturday, the extended side of my mom's family gathers at Grandma's. Mom's siblings with their spouses are inside the white, two-story abode amidst their childhood stomping grounds. Outside, the school-age siblings and cousins between the ages of four and thirteen bask in the sun under blue skies, aglow with blushed skin. We kids can hear the adults' indistinct chatter and laughter lilt through the open screens and out to us on an easy breeze. The tones, resonance, and cadence of the adults' rising and falling voices give away who is speaking, but not what is being said.

Gangly-limbed boys and girls take over the backyard between the terrace stone wall and the alleyway. "Batter up," Bigbro says, or in this case, kicker up would be more appropriate. He recruits us in a three-on-three kickball game. Two large sticks suffice as first and third bases, and home plate is the loose rock at the base of the low, stone retaining wall. Second base is the smooth stone face under the lilac tree, grown beyond a bush for decades, never cut back. Its blooms waft lavender sweetness in the air. We kids are unsupervised, save for Great-Grandma snagging the laundry off the clothesline, located in what would be the stadium seats of the third baseline.

Teams are a fair mix of ages and genders. My brothers (Lilbro, seven and Bigbro, thirteen) sport matching bowl cuts, brunette and blond respectively, compliments of my mother. Cousin Lynn (eight), with shoulder-length dishwater blonde hair, joins them in the field. Up to kick is my team: me, age ten with light blonde bangs and pigtails, Eric, also ten with cropped, unruly reddish-brown curls, and Ann, nearly eight with her Dorothy Hamill do. It is Ann's turn to kick, but as is often the case, she is tired and doesn't want to play anymore. She slumps under the shade of a maple tree with her little sister, our youngest cousin, Sue, aged four. Sue, being both the smallest and recovering from congenital hip dysplasia, gleefully leads cheers on the sidelines for both teams. Ann is content to share Sue's shady spot away from the playing field. Despite our peer pressure "please" pleas, Ann remains rooted to the lawn ledge. With uneven teams, Bigbro declares, "I'll be the all-time pitcher for both teams."

"I have a better idea," I announce and holler over my shoulder, "Come on, Great-Grandma! You can make the teams even. Play on my team." I beg her to join. Her silvery bun glistens while her skin-draped arms dismantle the hanging sunbaked bedding, long since dripped dry.

"Oh, no," she chuckles, "I don't know how to play."

"It's easy, Grandma. You just kick the ball and run around the bases," I reassure her.

She continues to protest through giggles that hint possibility, as one by one, the calico sheets appear to dance off the clothesline and fold themselves into a wicker basket by her simple sleight of hand. These pastel linens match what I imagine would have befit the bed of the Easter Bunny, before being faded by age and wear.

"It will be fun," I insist as my hand grasps hers and leads her away from the nearly nostalgic chore, and the kids chime in agreement.

Her laughter drifts nearer the playing field as she takes off her apron and drapes it over the neatly folded laundry pile. Great-Grandma always wears dresses, no matter the occasion. She owns neither shorts nor slacks, not to mention sneakers. If chores warrant a red-print dress and stout, black heels, so must a sporting event.

Through her chuckles she insists, "I've never played sports, not even as a young girl. I don't know why in Heaven's name I should start now, not at my age. I'm eighty-seven, you know!"

"I know, Great-Grandma. You're not too old, and it's easy. You just kick the ball and run around the bases." I can feel her light-hearted nature and the kid within her giving in to temptation. I coach her—one last rundown of the game's rules—and she steps up to the plate.

Bigbro rolls the large, swirl-blue, dime-store ball right under her high-kick step. "Strike one!"

Her chuckles rise into chortles. Lilbro and Lynn instinctively move closer infield as our team shouts encouraging words.

Bigbro pitches the ball along the grass a bit slower and... *bam!* Grandma's foot makes contact! The indigo orb sails over Bigbro's head and its trajectory sends Lilbro into the alley after it.

"Run, Great-Grandma, run!" my team cheers.

"Oh! Okay!" she shakes free of her amazed daze and takes off running—straight to third base! Perhaps my directions should have been more specific. I did say just kick the ball and run around the bases, and she did. Grandma continues her clockwise jaunt to the lilac tree (second base), whooping with deep, belly guffaws that would rival Santa. "Ho-ho-ho, ho-ho-ho, ho-ho-ho…." Meanwhile, the fielders purposely miss their attempts to throw her out at each base. The contralto "ho-ho-ho," is a continuous chorus as she rounds first and completes her reverse home run to an eruption of cheers.

Breathless, girlish with glee, she collapses to sit on the stone ledge and falls back into the velvety greenness behind, "I haven't had that much excitement in years!" Her grin presses deeply past her flushed cheeks as her hazel eyes reflect the sky above, a light hue of robin's egg blue. We all sing her praises about how good she is at kickball and encourage her to go again. "Oh, that's enough for one day," she declares. "Help me up." And no persuading convinces her otherwise.

All seven of us raise her up from the lawn to the heave count of three, Great-Grandma smooths her dress, reties her apron, and goes back to plucking her wooden clothespins, still grinning. By this time Ann is both rested and roused enough to play again and our teams are righted for another round, minus Great-Grandma.

Great-Grandma's kickball stats: recruited and retired the same day, one at-bat, one strike, one home run (on errors),… and one belly laugh for the All-Stars Hall of Fame.

I love my great-grandma to pieces, and she's my favorite person in the world. Our connection is so integral, that I know the moment she dies.

I am fifteen, at home in my messy teenage bedroom, fast asleep in my bed. In the middle of the night, my dreaming shifts into a surreal vision. In the vision, I am instantly transported from my bedroom to my grandmother's house and into Great-Grandma's bedroom. Her lifeless body lies before me in her bed, and it's clear to me that she is dead. It feels too visceral for it not to be true. At the instant of this realization, I am transported back to my bedroom with a jolt. I shoot straight up in bed and can feel the devastation of her death like a knife in my gut. My beloved great-grandmother's human form no longer shares the planet with me. I wail long and hard into my pillow, muffling my cries and quieting my grief, to keep from waking the household. It seems to take hours for my tears to subside. The remainder of the night, I toss and turn, eventually falling into a fitful sleep from distressed exhaustion.

Immediately in the morning, I rush to call my grandma on the phone to confirm the dreadful news I know I will hear.

"Great-Grandma is just fine," Grandma says casually. "I just took her morning toast and tea up to her, and she's dunking it and nibbling it as usual."

To my shock and disbelief, I wonder how can Great-Grandma be fine? How can she be eating breakfast? I saw her last night. She was dead. I know she was dead. How can I be so wrong about something that I am so certain of? There is no phone upstairs in their house, so I cannot hear Great-Grandma's voice for myself, but I do not doubt my grandma's word.

For the past six months, Great-Grandma has been relegated to the upstairs of the house, mostly staying in her bedroom, so she can access the only bathroom in her home, just at the end of the hall of the second story. At age ninety-two, she can no longer go up and down the stairs safely, not even with help. She has forgotten who all of my other relatives are, even thinking her own daughter is a staff person, working at whatever nursing home she now occupies. She is confused as to why she never sees any other residents, not realizing she is still living in her own home, with her daughter, as she has for decades. Despite her confusion, she always knows and recognizes me, except for a brief encounter a couple of months ago.

On my former visit, I enter her bedroom, and she is sitting up in bed.

"Hi Great-Grandma," I announce myself with a smile and a peck on the cheek, our usual greeting.

"Who are you?" she asks innocently yet sincerely.

"It's me, Deborah, your great-granddaughter," I help myself to the black and white picture of me, as a two-year-old, framed on her bureau, and place it in her hands.

She peruses my face with her gaze, glancing back and forth between me and the picture, and then sighs, "Oh, yes, of course. I know you. How silly of me," she laughs, and both of us are relieved.

The furnishings in Great-Grandma's bedroom are antique, dark walnut, sturdy, turn-of-the-century pieces from her father's furniture store. I am most fascinated by on old trunk stored under the window, home to family heirlooms, treasures that include formal full-length gloves, feathery and lacy folding hand fans, doilies and needlework, and a curious, tissue-lined box holding Great-Grandma's long, braided, brunette hair, cut off and saved, for what purpose I never ask.

On her night table sits an always-ticking clock that keeps me awake whenever I sleep over. It seems I can even hear it in my dreams. Shiny and silver, it's a round windup-style alarm clock, with bells on top that ring us awake in a startling clatter, or so I think when I jump to the ceiling first thing in the morning. I long to hear its rhythmic ticking again in the morning after my vision.

Hanging up the phone with Grandma, and despite her reassurance, I implore my mom to drive me to see Great-Grandma, as soon as possible. It takes forever to arrive at her house. Once inside, I scurry up the steps two at a time to her room, and silently gasp upon seeing her. It is just as my grandma said. Here is Great-Grandma, sitting up in bed, setting her magazine aside to smile at me. She is not dead. She is every bit as much alive as I am.

We exchange our usual greetings with a kiss on the cheek. I am mesmerized to be sitting on my great-grandma's bed, staring at her face-to-face as if it is some kind of miracle. We chat in our usual easy manner about everything and nothing at all, while the clock's ticking counts off the minutes of our time together.

After a natural pause in our conversation, she intently locks eyes with mine and says, "You know... I died last night."

I nod, tears brimming my eyes, and reply, "I know, Great-Grandma." I feel a wave of relief and grief intermingled. I am relieved that my knowing is spot-on. I am grieved that my knowing is spot-on.

She went on to describe the heaven she visited, a joyous place, and all her friends and relatives were there. Jesus was there too, and she saw and talked to him and felt only love. She insists she is happy to go back, and she doesn't want me to be sad for her. Then she intentionally pauses, reconnecting our mutual gaze, and says, "I just came back to tell you goodbye."

What an incredible gift! She must have felt with our soul connection how devastated I was at her passing from this world, even though she didn't say so, and returned to give me reassurance and peace. Mission accomplished! Instantly my fear of dying vanishes. And while I am truly happy for her, as she wishes, I am still sad for me, having to wait the rest of my life to see her again.

I don't want to leave her bedside. I know this is our last earthly encounter. I know she will never again twist the key on the bedside clock. The ticks will wind down, falling silent. But eventually, I have to go. We both know it's time. We exchange hugs and kisses and I-love-yous, our parting gifts to each other. She has a twinkle in her eye as I leave her room.

My eyes, instead, spill over with tears, and I can't keep myself from crying as I flee down the flight of stairs and out the front door. Mom and Grandma call after me, "Is everything all right? Is Great-Grandma okay?"

"Yes, everything is fine," I say through my tears, already outside. Grandma, not convinced, hurries back upstairs to see if anything's amiss.

"She's fine," Grandma's voice trails down the stairwell to my mom, who looks confused.

"I told you, everything is fine. Let's just go home," my voice strains into an unintended plea. I can't explain my tears to her satisfaction, but she indulges my request for the second time today.

We bid Grandma a hasty farewell. She waves to us from the curbside as Mom steers the car away from her childhood home, Great-Grandma tucked within, and turns from the city streets toward our country road home.

Later that same night, merely hours after my momentous visit with her, Great-Grandma dies peacefully in her sleep.

*As time went on we stumbled
Through something of a life.
Then Daddy flew the cuckoo's nest
Leaving us behind.
And Mom was left to clean up
Broken pieces that he made.
I guess it became easier
For him to...
    go away.*

Chapter 11

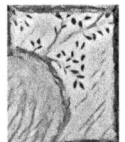

A Rudderless Young Adulthood

Two weeks before my high school senior year begins, Dad takes off. He disappears. He's gone. For good this time. Leaving behind empty drawers, empty closets, and an empty hole that held his toothbrush. I can't believe he did it! My surprise is that Dad wears his restlessness like a seasonal jacket, fetching it when a brooding storm disturbs his mind, donning it as he ventures out in the wind to clear his head, shedding it upon return when his foul mood blows over, hanging it on a coat hook, ready for the next time storm fronts loom.

    I am first aware of his urge to flee in third grade. Twirling in swirls on the elementary playground after school, I amuse myself while waiting for my dad to collect me. My piano lesson with Mrs. Carson is today, and Dad's driving me to her house. The other kids have scurried home after the dismissal bell, so it's just me left to play on my own. I meander around the paved open area, looking up at the sky, daydreaming about what it would be like to be a bird, to be able to fly. I flap my arms and spiral around, pretending to soar, rising far, far away.

Dad spots me mid-flight. He strides toward me, having parked the car along the curb beyond the tall chain-link fence that designates the school property. I fly to him, arms still flapping, and he stops me, saying, "Let me talk with you for a minute. I want to ask you something." The grasp of his hand holding mine clips my wings, grounding my flight, landing me back on earth. He guides me into a slow step beside him, reentering the playground. His voice is deliberate, the tension in his tone suggesting he is about to relay something important.

"How would you feel if I left?" Dad asks. I stop and stare at him. He searches my face for a reaction. I am instantly struck by the adult conversation we are having and that I am too young to be consulted on such a serious matter.

He continues, "What if I didn't live with you and Mom and the boys anymore? What would you think about that?" I also keenly sense that he wants me to erupt into a fit of tears, crying out, *No, No, No,* and pleading for him, *Stay. Please stay.* If I do this, I know I will make the decision for him, easing his guilt as he uses me as an excuse to stay, telling himself and me he will remain to keep me happy. I will not let him get away with using me.

Instead, I exude calm and poise, and my reply may seem wise beyond my years to someone else, but not to me, "I think you should do whatever is best for you. If it is best for you to stay, then stay. If it is best for you to leave, then leave. You should do whatever makes you happy." My words and demeanor thump him between the eyes. The tearful protest he was counting on doesn't materialize. He has no plan B.

Dad backpedals a bit, stammering, "Well… I guess I'll probably stay…. I just wanted to know how it would make you feel."

"I would be sad, but I would be okay. My friend Jenny's parents are divorced, and she's fine."

He cocks his head at me in a shrugging "huh" kind of way, rethinking what he thought he knew about me, sizing me up as a peer rather than as a child. There was nothing more to say. We drove off to my piano lesson as if our conversation had never occurred, as if it were any other day.

I do recall about six months after our poignant playground conversation and every six months thereafter, that a monumental tsunami surged, provoking his dramatic exodus from the ranch house, hollering as the door bangs, "I'm leaving! I might not come back!" He careens away but predictably shifts gears, returning after a matter of hours or maybe a whole day later. But the car always rolls him back home, in time for supper before a second sunset.

Not this time. His leaving prior to my senior year, at the close of my seventeenth summer, is different. There is no precipitating fight between my parents, no storming out. He vanishes unannounced, covertly.

Arriving home from church one Sunday morning, a note, penned in Dad's hand, perches on my bed pillow. I read that my dad is unhappy and needs to find himself. In order to do that, he can't handle the responsibility of being a husband or a father right now.

It's nothing I've done. Oh, and he loves me, and to please forgive him. My mom and my brothers each get their own, similar letters. A stoic void hangs over the house, a missing suitcase, a bedroom closet half empty, bare drawers, and absent shoes—he's gone, the scent of aftershave lingering in the air.

Mom gazes out the bedroom window, in a distant stare, with tears in her eyes, her note folded in her hand. I reach out and hold her in an awkward hug, an attempt to comfort her in a pose unfamiliar between us. For the first time ever, I utter the unspoken words that have forever hung in silence in the air surrounding our family of five, now four, "I love you, Mom."

"Thank you, Deborah," she reciprocates with her own unpracticed, "I love you, too."

Growing up, I never doubt that my parents love me, even during my teenage rantings when I declare that I must be adopted because my real parents would never treat me this way. It's baffling why the emotion of love is assumed but not expressed in words, hinted at but not mentioned, tiptoed around but not spoken aloud. Instead, love is expressed in dance lessons and piano teachers, in summer church camp and family vacations, in signed permission slips and school program attendance, in holiday celebrations, and especially birthday parties.

Birthdays in our family manifest in shindigs, and the birthday star declares the theme by selecting a cake design. Amongst her cookbooks, Mom keeps catalogs of cutout cakes for us kids to choose from, which include color pictures of the finished creations and step-by-step instructions on how to make them.

I recall perusing the pages with excitement, finding just the right cake to celebrate my upcoming birthday party. For my party, when I turn four, I choose Mother Goose, and for the age of five, I pick Raggedy Ann. My older brother selects a train, and my younger brother opts for a clown, and by the time we all reach the age of 18, I wonder, between the three of us, if there is any cake pictured left unmade. Proof of each cake, for both me and my brothers, is tucked away in a photo album on a shelf in Mom's organized collection of pictures, commemorating all family celebrations in order of occurrence. Mom recreates each cake perfectly, buys complementary napkins and decorations to match, and sets up the idyllic display in the formal dining room, complete with a lacy tablecloth and a crystal punchbowl.

The relatives gather to mark the occasions of me being a year older. Both sides of my extended and intergenerational family play the continuous cycle of party characters, who are also a year older than the year before. Fashions and hairstyles change, but the guest list retains the same assortment, kids, teens, middle-agers and elders. The premier cake, mixed nuts, butter mints, and fizzy red punch, along with Hallmark cards and dazzling wrapped gifts, mark the anniversary of my arrival on the planet. Only Santa can rival the anticipation and excitement of my birthday party. In years when my age turns an even number, Mom splurges on an additional friends party, and an extra round of "Happy Birthday" is sung by my besties before we eat vanilla ice cream and chocolate cupcakes with sprinkles, then battle for prizes playing Twister and musical chairs.

I guess Dad will miss my eighteenth birthday this year. His parents, in-laws to my mother, stop by two days after my dad's disappearance, reassuring my mother and us kids that they do not approve of their son abandoning us, and that they will continue to be present as part of our family life, like always. None of us, not even Grandpa and Grandma, know where he's gone.

Starting my senior year of high school is extra weird because of Dad's leaving, in that Dad teaches at my high school. His room is in the industrial arts wing, so I rarely see him in the hallways and never elect to take his classes. Our classmates dub the handful of us (that qualify) as "teacher's kids," and I capitalize on this perk. When there's early morning marching band practice, I snag a ride with Dad. If I miss the bus after school, I catch a ride home with Dad. If I forget my lunch money, I knock on the teacher's lounge door, and after choking back the billow of cigarette smoke, I score cash from Dad. If the musical production needs stage set pieces from the high school across town, my friends and I snatch my dad's van keys during study hall and fetch them. Being a teacher's kid also means the faculty members know me, the staff workers know me, the principals know me, and all the kids in the school know my dad, and they like him, with his reputation of being kind of goofy in a good way.

But this year, haunted hallways echo with the unknown. I wonder if Lilbro feels this way too. He's just starting his freshman year of high school, newly exploring the senior high experience, the untraversed building layout, and the novel label, "teacher's kid."

The three of us occupy the same space, all day, five days a week, but in different areas. It's weird knowing my dad works within adjacent walls but not knowing where he lives after school. Will I have a chance run-in with him in the hallway? If I do, what will I say, or what will he say? Will we just pass each other by without saying anything? I purposefully avoid his end of the building. I don't want to see him. The question marks shadow me throughout each school day.

A couple of months into the semester, a fellow band underclassman makes a casual comment about my dad living in his father's rental building, as if it's common knowledge. This is news to me. "Oh, I'm sorry, I thought you knew." He jots down the address and the apartment number. When I steel my nerves, I ambush my dad with an unannounced visit.

Dad opens the door wide, and his chin drops into an astonished smile. "How did you find me?"

"I know your landlord's son. He told me you live here."

He laughs, genuinely surprised but delighted to see me, "Come in, come in. I can't believe you're here."

He ushers me into the dumpy abode. Clearly, the band kid's father is a slumlord. "It's all I can afford," my dad shrugs self-consciously.

"Let me show you around!" His giddiness resembles a college kid living off-campus for the first time, his apartment barely larger than a dorm room. He gives me the grand tour, pointing to and naming the obvious areas of the sparsely furnished living quarters as I shuffle my feet, swiveling round in place to view.

Gesturing to the dining table, two chairs wide, he invites, "Come, sit down. Tell me about the family. How's everybody doing?"

We squeeze into the chairs. I'm stunned but manage to mumble. "We're fine."

"Good, that's good. I've been cooking for myself. Mostly just Hamburger Helper and Dinty Moore Beef Stew, but I'm getting by...."

Distracted by my thoughts, I barely hear him as he continues prattling on about himself. How can he be so casual? Why is he so happy? It's not just being pleased to see me—he prefers his squalor to being with our family, to living in our home. Where's his apology for vanishing, his guilt about abandoning us, his remorse for destroying our family? It dawns on me that Dad is clueless to the reality that his leaving devastated the rest of us, individually and collectively. I don't have the gumption to burst his bubble. It took all my stamina to brace myself to see him.

"Well, I should go...."

I need to get out. Away from him.

"Oh sure, you've got things to do." He gets up and holds open the door for me. "Thanks for stopping by. Come back anytime!" he smiles and waves as I head toward the family car.

"Okay, Dad. Bye!" I dash down the sidewalk to the curb, weary of his presence, allowing him to bask in his imaginary dream state that all's right with the world. I observe him shrinking in the rearview mirror, dissolving to dust, as I wind the car along the four-mile route, bawling the whole way home.

Before my dad's hasty departure, I am on track to marry my high school boyfriend, Jack. There is no formal proposal, just a promise ring and mutual understanding that we are heading in that direction. We both want to be teachers, he high school history and me elementary music. I like the idea of having identical schedules and summers off to raise our future family. Even though I notice parallel dysfunctions in our relationship and that of my parents, I accept it as the normal, healthy discourse of a long-term couple. Now, with my parents separated, I'm having second thoughts. My thoughts are so strong that I concoct a plot to give Jack an excuse to break up with me by kissing another boy. But after I do that and confess, Jack wants to work things out instead. Plan foiled. I will not make the same mistake as my parents by marrying my high school sweetheart. I cannot save my mother, but I can save myself. I break up with Jack.

Dad is overly fair in his divorce settlement with Mom, presumably out of guilt. I am not present at the meetings, but hear that he contests nothing, offers my mom the house in lieu of alimony, the nicer car, full custody of Lilbro and me, child support, and voluntarily forfeiture of his visitation rights. Bigbro is already an adult, on his own in the world. The uncontested, out-of-court settlement takes about six months from start to finish. Both parties sign the papers in the spring before I graduate and, just like that, the 24-year marriage is over. The divorce, final.

My dad's search for himself turns out to be a hoax. I discover that his over-eagerness to swiftly settle the divorce terms is a ploy to conceal a lie, a lie which, if discovered, could complicate the divorce proceedings with Mom. Dad keeps a girlfriend in a neighboring state, a woman he met while attending an extended-stay continuing education class in her town the previous summer. The two have coupled covertly ever since. Their schemed wedding date is early summer, after I graduate—devised preemptively, the plans pre-dating the divorce. Did I mention his betrothed has a five-year-old son? So much for not being able to handle the responsibilities of being a husband and father! He didn't find himself, he found someone else.

When I confront him about this lie from his parting note and point out the obvious contradiction, he sounds like a juvenile caught breaking the rules. He spins a life-and-death scenario, where he was desperate to leave a marriage that was killing him, and he did what he needed to do and said what he needed to say to save himself.

Mr. and Mrs. Dad's Second Marriage is made official in the bride's hometown in the neighboring state, on her family's farm at an outdoor ceremony. I attend, reasoning that it would hurt my dad more for me to *not* be there than it would hurt me to go. I question if my reasoning proves true. While mingling with the bride's side of the family, I uncover that the whole wedding is a farce based on a lie. Clearly, from speaking with the guests related to my dad's new wife, including her parents, I discover they all are under the same misimpression—that my father was divorced long ago, before the newlyweds began seeing each other—and isn't it wonderful that they both get a second chance at love? No harm! No foul! Happy new life! They all just love my dad. Of course, they do. Everybody does. Everybody always has. In public arenas, he shapeshifts into an entertaining people-pleaser, knowing his audience, playing for laughs, performing in ways that garner applause. My dad and his new wife lied to every person present. Why wouldn't they? I know I am the most unhappy person at this "blessed" event.

Newly in love, I'm certain my second long-term boyfriend, Shawn, and I will be together forever. It's still my senior year in high school, but only his sophomore year. In true boyfriend fashion, Shawn is my date for Senior Prom and goes to all my peer graduation parties with me, then stands beside me at my own. We spend every minute of the summer we can together, knowing time is accelerating toward my leaving home for college, both of us dreading our separation.

Two friends from my graduating class will join me in the full-day's drive from our hometown to the private school, prided for its quality music program. The trio of us register as music majors, all earning music scholarships, mine funding the cost of voice and piano instruction. My nervous excitement builds as I eagerly anticipate this next adventure, leaving the nest, testing my wings, learning to fly solo.

In the first week of college, I am reduced to a sparrow among songbirds, a chorister among divas, a talentless hack among polished musicians. My voice audition lands me in the lowest choir. An original song I write and sing with a friend does not even qualify for the freshman showcase talent show. My high school days of starring roles in musicals and getting number one rankings in voice solo contests are over. It appears I have already peaked. I had consoled myself over my devastating failure to make the All-State Chorus my senior year by saying it was an unlucky fluke. Perhaps not. My musical gifts display as childish here, my compositions as bland and simple, my voice as strained and wispy, my musicianship as basic and lacking.

What happened to that special something the talent scout from California mentioned a mere four years ago? In addition to having to accept that my skills are remedial compared to my advanced peers, my required music coursework proves beyond me. Sight Singing class is worse than sight-reading a piano score. Unlike a piano key, my voice does not automatically sing the note I see on the page; unlike my piano fingering, my voice doesn't leap to the correct interval; and, unlike my private lesson, I practice with an audience of classmates, screeching out my mistakes for all to hear.

Just as Sight Singing class drains my confidence, Music Theory class saps my passion. The beauty of music as art is wrecked through intellectual reductionism—which turns intricate chord progressions into sterile math equations and deconstructs masterpieces for the purpose of mental analysis—as if music was meant to be rational. What good is it for my mind to understand music logically when I've always played by heart what I felt in my soul? I'm barely managing

Cs in the core curriculum. After my first semester of enduring this academic humiliation, I can't picture myself suffering through three and a half more years of these same classes with the content increasing in difficulty. My dream of becoming an elementary music schoolteacher fades away from me like a long decrescendo into a ritardando. It is heartbreaking to realize these advanced skill obstacles go beyond anything I would be expected to teach in an elementary music classroom setting.

Part of my financial aid package includes a requirement for work-study. I am assigned to the cafeteria and rotate between the various tasks: dishwashing, serving, and busing tables. I don't mind working. I've rung up department store purchases for shoppers as a cashier since the age of 16 and am still on the schedule for college breaks and summers. I do mind the snarky nickname the wealthier coeds call the student workers like me—"wusses"—their pronunciation of WS, the abbreviation for work-study. I know it's a slam referring to a weakling. It sounds like an antiquated '50s insult from the TV show *Happy Days* I watched with my family while growing up. I didn't experience cliques and snobbery in my high school, unlike the '80s teen movie depictions. We had teen packs centered around what people liked to do, but they overlapped with interchanging members. One could be both a jock and a music geek, both a cheerleader and a science nerd, and no one fussed. I thought the movies that depicted these social class distinctions of my generation to be

Hollywood exaggerations. However, the hotshots at my college were laughable in emulating these fictional characters in real life. Who invented this variation on the term *wuss*, and why would anyone actually use it? But someone did. And they do. A lot.

One of my dorm roommates is a Hollywood caricature rich kid without knowing it. On weekends, she invites me to spree with her at the nearest shopping mall, and I always decline. One day she takes offense and accusingly asks me, "Why do you never want to go shopping with me? Don't you like me?"

"Yes, I like you. I just don't have any money to buy anything." I answer honestly. "It's no fun to go shopping and come back empty-handed."

"Oh, well, just call your parents and have them put money on your credit card," she responds as if the problem is solved.

"I don't have a credit card," I respond, "and even if I did, my parents don't have extra money to give me."

She looks perplexed, trying to resolve the dissonance in her brain that can't comprehend a reality so different from her own. Then she has a lightbulb moment and says, "Oh, yeah! You're a wuss. I've seen you in the cafeteria," connecting the dots. "Oh, well that makes sense." She seems content that I like her and have good reason for declining her shopping invite. I don't like her at the moment. She doesn't think she's using the word wuss in a derogatory way, not realizing that the word itself is offensive rather than a simple descriptor. She is clueless that she's just insulted me. The upside is, she never asks me to go shopping again.

There is a January term, only a month long, that I opt out of to work my cashier job at home and have an extended Christmas break with my long-distance boyfriend Shawn, now a high school junior. I leave for the second semester that starts in February, and by March, I am back home again, aged 19, this time medically discharged for the semester with a case of mononucleosis.

How have I contracted a kissing disease when the only person I have kissed is Shawn, and he remains healthy? Still, I am exhausted and sleep throughout the day, sporting swollen glands and a sore throat. I know that I will not return to the posh music campus next term. The financial aid package decidedly alters because my mom returns to work, and I am offered student loans instead of grants, with terms too huge to consider reasonable to repay on an eventual teacher's salary. Abandoning my elementary school music teacher career, I opt for the next best thing—becoming an elementary classroom teacher.

Part-time by the middle of April, full-time by the end of May, I stand at my department store register again, donning my standard-issue smock and scanning the tags to rhythmic beeps as swim towels and flip flops roll down the conveyor belt. When summer starts, I favor vast exclusive times with Shawn, as he's freed from school, and I conjure what to do in the fall. There's a small college just across the state line that I can attend at the in-state tuition rate. My dad earned his master's degree there, and they allow children of graduates the lowest rates, regardless of where they live. I'll be close enough to see Shawn on the weekends and can continue my education, a bit delayed.

Who can recall the discourse between my mom and me during my nineteenth summer? We engage in verbal tugs-of-war over disputed house rules, we dig in our heels over mutual turf, we set boundaries ablaze and extinguish the flames with stomping tirades, with buckets of tears. The foreground is me jostling for adult footing while acting like a child, and my mom treating me like a child while acting like one herself.

The backdrop is the abrupt dismantling of our family, that was neither discussed as it was happening, nor is discussed now, except during a few sessions of family counseling my brothers and I attend with her. The sessions suddenly cease after the therapist draws a diagram of our family dynamic, a circle with Mom at the center, and arrows of the rest of us pointing out and away from her. Our family pattern on the surface is clean, glazed, and polished for a perfect reflection, creating a pristine sheen for public viewing, but we never examine whatever ugliness may lurk underneath. Our conflicts, never resolved, remain contentious as we fight atop an emotional burial ground of unmarked graves. By the time I'm ready to move to campus at the new college, I'm exhausted, ready to be done battling with Mom, and I can't wait to escape. I know it is not just her. We are toxic together, each bringing out the worst in the other. I'm sure she will be just as relieved to have me gone.

On moving day, Mom assumes that she is going with me, that the two of us, mother and daughter, are going to nest me into my new dorm room together, as if the awful tension of the summer never happened. I can't endure this false pretense, her enacting the happy facade, dismissing the stress of us being at odds in order to put a good face on the next chapter of my life. (It doesn't occur to me that this is her way of showing her love for me, her way of wishing me well.)

Mom is in the driveway, getting the car ready for packing. "Get your stuff, Deborah, it's time to start loading the car."

"I'm not loading the car, Mom. I'm waiting for Shawn. We're taking his car. He's taking me to school."

The scene goes as well as I expected, which is not well at all. I try to let her down easy, but she won't let me. Mom won't abide my decision, she won't let me go without her, not without another verbal fight. I wish she would yield before I end up saying something awful. She doesn't. I do. "I need a fresh start, and that fresh start does not include you," I cringe as the syllables escape my lips.

Her eyes brim with tears, but she finally relents. Am I drawing a clear boundary that she cannot accept? Am I just being cruel? Am I like my father? I don't even know if the answers to these questions matter, as I've stabbed her in the heart. It's as if my freedom comes with the cost of wounding her. Would it really be so terrible for me to let her do the mother/daughter thing the way she wants to, even if I'm not up for it? For whatever reason, and I don't know why, my answer is yes, it would be so terrible. It just isn't in me to surrender. Not today.

Arriving at my new campus home, I see the familiar buildings dotted between connecting sidewalks crisscrossing the lawns, the slant-roofed auditorium where our high school swing choir competed, the windowed music hall of my clarinet solo contest, the brick medical arts studio where my dad's youngest sister, only ten years older than I, made a ceramic cast of my teeth for her dental hygienist course. It's a sunny move-in Saturday afternoon, with classes starting on Wednesday morning.

My first trip to the cafeteria Saturday evening reminds me of high school. The lunch tables are just the same—the portable kind that unfolds in the middle and spreads out on wheels to provide picnic-bench-style seating. The room is large and open, with a wood floor, akin to the high school gym we used as a temporary lunchroom midday between PE classes, only here the room has windows, a low ceiling, and is a designated dining area. Carrying my self-serve, a la carte feast on my tray, I spy a cluster of my high school classmates I haven't seen since graduation, milling around the drink station with their own trays. Our reunion is brief, perfunctory, with a hey-nice-to-see-you, and a see-you-around, tossed my way as they move on to sit elsewhere without an invitation for me to join them. Instead, I plop my tray down with some girls I have just met from my dorm floor.

Everything about this scene is wrong. I don't want to be here. I don't belong. Something inside me screams to leave. The girls chatting next to and across from me sound as if they are in an echo chamber, and their faces blur long and wide, like adjusting the horizontal and vertical settings on a tube TV. I chalk it up to first day jitters and contribute nothing to the conversation except weak smiles and head nods. Surely things will look better in the morning after a good night's sleep. It's been an eventful day, with the horrid parting from Mom this morning, the tearful driving away of Shawn this afternoon, though for not so long and not so far, and settling into a new dormitory this evening.

My roommate seems nice. I'm grateful that she's a sophomore and not an incoming freshman, that we've both done this away-from-home college-thing before, that we have something in common. I soon get the impression I appear frivolous to her, like the way I viewed my let's-go-shopping roommate last year, as she watches me unpack my clothes and hang them in the wardrobe. My suitcase had remained zipped throughout the day, waiting for Shawn to leave. I reserved as much quality time with Shawn as possible, not wasting our time with mindless tasks I could do on my own once he'd gone.

A sizable portion of my cashier's paycheck I spend on new outfits for the school year. Fresh start. Fresh style. I embrace my new career choice with pieces to look the part of a teacher, knowing my first semester, I will be shadowing in an actual elementary school classroom. I choose bold primary colors for quilted skirts, blouses, sweaters, belts, and shoes, that I can mix and match into a variety of dressy, yet comfortable attire. The price tags still dangle from the items.

"Your parents bought you all new clothes for school?" My roommate seems genuinely curious, yet her subtle tone implies I'm spoiled.

"No, I purchased them myself with my own money from working my job as a cashier," I reply matter-of-factly, without defense, as I continue to hang and fold. I align the alike colors, yellows, blues, and reds, satisfied with my coordinated arrangement, as they now drape neatly in place.

"And you've never worn any of them before now?" she asks the obvious, with a tone that implies I'm ridiculous.

"No, I am saving them for this special occasion. I didn't want to wear them out before school started." My splurge to make myself feel confident has backfired into insecure vanity within this short conversation. Why didn't I take the tags off at home? Would we even be having this conversation if there was no way to tell these clothes were brand new? I feel as lame as her judgment suggests. Just who am I trying to impress? I don't think I'm trying to impress anyone, but now I second-guess myself. Looking at my roommate on her top bunk behind me through the mirrored closet door, I find it glaringly obvious that this new wardrobe is an attempt to cover my insecurities with a stylish distraction, and this roommate who has known me for merely a few hours sees right through me. "It's no big deal," I say, and hastily begin snatching the tags, one by one, tossing them into the trash.

My roomie sees she has flustered me and softens a bit. "I'm sorry," she offers, and says, "It just seems weird to me, that's all. I've never seen so many new clothes all at once before except in a store." I appreciate her attempt to make me feel better and try to hide that she has shaken me.

"Yeah, me neither. I just thought it would be nice for a change," and the matter is dropped.

Sunday, I wake up in my dorm room's bottom bunk and don't feel any better about being here. This is way beyond the Shadow Monster. The refrain seems to be coming from the universe. The booming voice reverberates, "You don't belong here! You don't belong here!" Not only do I hear it echoing in my head, I feel it resounding in my body, quaking within my core, yanking at my soul. I look around to see if others can hear it too, the words are so blaring. It is not a message of self-insecurity, indicating to me that I am not fitting in with these people at this school. This is a message of, "You are in the wrong latitude and longitude on the planet! Correct your coordinates!" That's the accurate, "You don't belong here," translation.

This is not first-day jitters, or second-day jitters, or even starting-over jitters. This is not the Shadow Monster speaking in its muffled somatic ways. This is a clear warning from something stronger than anything on this earthly plain. It's not scary as much as it is definite. The trajectory of my future will skew if I stay. I must depart to prevent some cosmic flight plan from irreversibly altering. It would be hard to believe if it weren't happening to me, but it is, and I have no choice but to listen. The registrar's office opens at 8:00 a.m. on Monday. I will go first thing in the morning and withdraw from school. As instantly as I make this decision, the booming voice stops. The dead silence is equally alarming.

Sunday afternoon, I swallow my pride and phone my mom. There is no plausible way to explain what I'm going through, that some divine intervention wants me to quit school. After my fretful insistence that I'm doing the right thing, she says, "Well, you can quit school if you want to, but you can't live here." I burned a bridge yesterday by not letting her move me into the dorms and my cruel "fresh start" comment. Now I am paying the price. Or does Mom think that if I have nowhere to go I will stay in school and tough it out? Either way, I'm floored by her response. The dial tone lingers in my ear as I hang up, scrambling for a backup plan. I call my dad.

    He and his second family have a newly constructed house in a subdivision being added to the west end of my hometown. My stepbrother, now six, will start kindergarten soon. The split-level house has a basement living area with half-windows, and a spare bedroom with its own full bathroom. There is room for me, but I hold little hope that his wife will agree, even though we have been cordial with each other in the year since the wedding. I have no choice but to ask my dad if I can live there temporarily until I figure out something else. He'll have to call me back, of course, after conferring with my stepmom, during which time he'll ask her what she thinks. Now I must wait in my dorm room for the phone to ring, because it is the age of only landlines, and I do not want to miss Dad's return phone call. I recline, unrelaxed in my bunk, shuffling names in my mind of who next to call if he says no.

    The phone rings sooner than I think, and I am pleasantly surprised. I can live in Dad's basement as long as I want, provided I pay $150 a month in rent, and with the caveat that, once I choose to leave, I won't be allowed back. My stepmom doesn't want the instability of people coming and going in her son's life. This sounds more than fair.

As we arrange, Dad picks up me and my repacked stuff on Monday at noon, after my registrar's visit to officially withdraw from school. The expense is two nights' lodging plus four meals, with an otherwise full refund.

College stats thus far: 0 for 2 colleges; 16 credit hours.

Second semester college freshman status: on leave. Again.

The rest of August and September go okay with the new basement living arrangement. The department store is more than happy to hire me back full-time, and there is ample time to spend with Shawn in his senior year of high school. At home, I keep mostly to myself on the lower level, popping up to make my meals and eating them downstairs.

I hear the discourse above of my stepbrother being strictly parented in ways I find unreasonably harsh. One morning on a school day, he gets up and helps himself to a bowl of cereal. In and of itself, this is fine; however, he opens a new box of a different flavor of cereal before finishing the old box already opened. Gruff adult rantings admonish the defenseless child, two against one, and I hear his pleas followed by the swats of my stepbrother's punishment—a spanking. I feel sorry for the poor guy, starting off his morning in tears before climbing onto the safety of the school bus. I pray his kindergarten teacher is nice to him.

October winds chill the autumn air, along with my living situation. The budding housing addition is rising out of a fallow cornfield. Surrounding the few finished homes, like ours, are vacant lots and new construction in various stages of completion. As the weather falls below freezing, the field mice, newly displaced, find preferable nests in the basement walls to keep warm. During the day, my living quarters remain relatively quiet. But all night long, scurrying and scritch-scratching in the walls keep me awake. I find it maddening. The newly purchased mouse traps are full and emptied daily but are not making a dent in the population. Dad refuses to call an exterminator, reasoning that there would be no way to get rid of all the mice, and that we would be paying for exterminating every mouse in the entire neighborhood. In my mind, if the mice were showing up on the upper level, he would call an exterminator, but so far, they have been content to remain down below, only affecting my living space. I start sleeping on the couch in the upstairs living room.

My mental state is as tenuous as ever, living in close quarters with the newly formed dysfunctional family that daily erupts into chaos over minor kid infractions. The inability to sleep comfortably in my own bed takes its toll. I am desperate to move but have nowhere else to go. I devolve into a basket case of tears when I am with Shawn, finally having his listening ear to unpack the stress of my living nightmare.

Shawn convinces his mom to give me temporary respite on the spare bed in her sewing room. I'm still paying my rent to my dad but sleeping at Shawn's. This arrangement becomes unacceptable to my stepmom, and she demands that I remove all of my belongings from her house or she will throw them in a dumpster. Dad stays out of it. Another plea from Shawn to his mom, and I can move a few of my things into Shawn's brother's bedroom. Shawn's brother has been away at college for the past several years and now has his own apartment in another city and only returns for visits, not to live.

"A few of my things" turns into "all my stuff," filling the bedroom from floor to ceiling with boxes and crates of my childhood treasures. By the time I finish, the small bedroom looks like an overstuffed college dorm room. I am pleased with how I manage to squeeze everything I own into the cramped space in a well-organized display of all my worldly possessions, hoping Shawn's mother won't mind. She peers into the room to check my progress. "What do you think?" I ask.

She replies solemnly and with great pause, "You don't want to know what I think." Her tact and restraint emphasize clearly that I have overstepped by completely taking over a room I am meant to be merely a guest in. She leaves a wake of thick tension in the air. It's a wake all too familiar to me. I have lived in a wake like this my whole life.

Every six months, my dad would cast this wake when he abruptly sped away in a huff, leaving the rest of us breathing shallowly, holding the surface tension of his unknown whereabouts and his indefinite return. Mom would carry on in his absence like nothing out of the ordinary was happening, as if everything was fine. When he returned without explanation of where he'd gone or what he'd been up to, no one questioned him or his behavior. The relief of having him home traded one surface tension for another—awaiting his next departure. Wakes of tension are the ocean waves in which I have learned to swim, though lately, it feels like I'm sinking.

I am aware that I am the only dysfunction in Shawn's otherwise functional family. They have a smooth and seamless way of being together. All I have to offer are my rough edges. The shroud of tension that envelops me is like that cloud of dust that always surrounds Pig-Pen in the *Peanuts* cartoons. It would seem I should finally be able to relax and release my protective armor, breathe easy and enjoy the peace. But this land of genuine calm is too unfamiliar to be comfortable, like a surreal dream that I am watching swirl around me but am not truly part of.

I celebrate my 20th birthday with my makeshift family—my high school senior boyfriend and his parents—as well as Christmas and the New Year. The quirky living situation begins to feel like a new normal to me, and I assume it will stay this way until Shawn graduates from high school and the two of us go off to college together.

One afternoon in late March, Mom calls, and it's not her usual check-in.

"I think it's time you move out of Shawn's house and come back home to live," she states.

"Why? I like it here, and Shawn and I will be leaving in six months for college anyway."

"I think it would be better for everyone if you lived here. I'd like you to come home."

"You're the one that kicked me out in the first place," I remind her, trying to mask my rising annoyance. "If you would have let me come home from college when I withdrew last fall, I would already be living with you, but you said, 'No.' Why would I want to live where I'm not wanted?"

"That was a long time ago. I do want you here now."

"I'd rather stay here, Mom." All the fights we waged last summer flash through my mind, the harsh words hurled, building up to our last dreadful parting that prevented our reunion. "I don't want to move all my stuff again before college. I can come home on school breaks once the semester starts. I think we both get along better when we don't live in the same house."

Mom sounds disappointed but relents adding, "Just know you are always welcome here, Deborah," before she hangs up the phone.

I cradle the receiver in disbelief. Her change of heart likely has more to do with her difficulty explaining my unconventional living situation to her church friends. I can't think of any other reason she'd want me home.

Shawn is the youngest of five children. His sister and brother-in-law live across town, and they visit the house frequently. On one particularly sunny Thursday in early April, I am alone in the house, as I have a day off from the department store, and both of Shawn's parents work while Shawn is at school. The brother-in-law shows up mid-morning and has news for me.

"Pack your things! You are moving out today—right now! You don't belong here. You have never belonged here. No one wants you here. You should have never moved in here in the first place! We're loading your things into my truck, and I'm taking you back to your mom's house immediately." His voice is terse, every word punctuated with emphasis, and he seems to relish his role as cruel evictor.

I am stunned, in shock as we two go through the swift motions, up and down the flight of stairs, emptying the house of my things, filling the truck, erasing all signs of my stay. In less than an hour, we pull into the driveway of the country ranch house, and there is my mom smiling and offering to help, as if this is a welcome turn of events, as if she never turned me away, as if the world is righting itself, as if the throw rug from Shawn's brother's room hadn't been yanked right out from under me.

Everyone knew but me. Shawn knew. His parents knew. My mom knew. Clearly, the brother-in-law and sister knew. All of them plotted and approved my abrupt relocation, picking the day and time to execute it, agreeing to ambush me, but not dictating the harsh manner of the resulting eviction. (When I cried to Shawn about the cruel words and brusque treatment, he was as appalled as I and told his parents. The brother-in-law took liberties in his zeal to remove me and was later reprimanded, with a forced apology to me in front of Shawn's family.) I always sensed that Shawn's brother-in-law didn't like me, and eviction day proved it.

Despite feeling betrayed, I keep dating Shawn in this return to a more traditional living style in two separate homes. I'm still the 20-year-old girlfriend attending the prom of an 18-year-old high school senior. Shawn and I apply and are both accepted into his school of choice, a state university. I look forward to our future move to the university setting where the age difference won't be so glaringly obvious and awkward for me.

A fresh adventure before us, Shawn and I kick off the fall university season together with new-found freedom, away from our families and living in neighboring dormitories on the east edge of campus. I may finally outrun my fumbled misstarts and jostled missteps as I tackle a few positives early in the season. Here, my vocal audition does score me a position in the top choir, and I am eligible for voice lessons, even though I am not a music major. An extra point: piano practice rooms are open 24 hours, which means I can play any time I want to for my own pleasure. The music building becomes my home away from the dorms.

I don't recognize any of the thousands of passing faces on campus except my boyfriend's. The past two years, I clung to Shawn for love, security, stability, and gave him every bit of my free time. But even when we shared a roof, I walked to work, and he drove to school, so our free time had breaks and interruptions from each other. Now, although we attend different classes throughout the day, our schedules otherwise align in identical open spaces, all the time. I assume Shawn and I will fill every free moment together. It starts out that way, but then Shawn has other plans.

I observe Shawn quickly bond with his three roommates, and they pal around together for eating meals, shooting hoops, and playing cards. I feel like an unwanted tag-a-long when I join them. My roommate, on the other hand, is a Greek-seeker who failed to get picked for her chosen sorority during rush week and resents being stuck in a dorm with me. Even more tragic, her boyfriend earns a fraternity pledge spot, and she's barred from attending frat parties, which are designed for schmoozing the sister sorority coeds. Greek system rules aren't made to be broken, and the biggest no-no is for a brother to date a girl outside of the Greek system. Before the semester ends, the boyfriend dumps my roommate, and my roommate dumps me, moving into an apartment off-campus. I luxuriate in a room to myself for the rest of the year.

The Monday after classes start, I sign up for mental health counseling at Student Services. In my first session, I am initially paired with a psychology graduate student who is supervised as part of his master's degree program. He seeks permission from me to record our sessions to be reviewed by his primary instructor. I know immediately that my troubles are beyond his beginner's training, but I play along and sign the release form so he can check off the required boxes.

The psychologist-in-training turns on the tape recorder, states his name, date, and time, and that this is our first session. "State your first name only, please."

"Deborah."

"And Deborah, have you agreed to have our session recorded and signed the permission slip? If so, say 'Yes.'"

"Yes."

"So, Deborah, what brings you in to see me today?" he settles back into listening mode.

I know my psychiatric diagnosis by rote, having been in the room when other doctors are consulting aloud about me and my case history, as if I am not present. "I have been receiving counseling and medication for depression for four years now and would like to continue to do so here at university. I have suicidal ideology, having an intense feeling of wanting to die, but have never acted on these feelings and have no plan to commit suicide."

Click! The grad student switches off the tape recorder. "That's all for today, Deborah. I am obligated to have you referred to a psychologist and am not qualified to talk with you any further. My scope of practice is limited to adjustment challenges from moving away from home and academic stress, things of that nature. I'll make sure the receptionist schedules an appointment for you with one of our staff professionals before you leave today." This is my record for the shortest counseling session ever, worthy of the *Guinness Book of World Records*, I think.

Between my weekly appointments with the staff psychologist and my daily dose of antidepressants, the Shadow Monster and I manage to trek off to classes and scribble homework assignments in the hustle and bustle of sidewalk mazes and the study lounges of inquiring minds. As for Shawn and me, the highs and lows of our romance match my mood swings. When I'm doing well, we're doing well. When I'm not so good, neither are we. In mere months the upswings stall, and we wallow in the murky downs. In the sea of our love, Shawn floats on a life preserver, but I swim without one and I cling to him for dear life, not letting go. Depression is like an anchor shackled to my ankle, and Shawn alone keeps me afloat. He resists my pulling him down, down, down, but cuts me loose to save himself. He must. Or he'll sink with me.

Suddenly, I am like my mother in the counselor's diagram, in the middle of the circle, with all the arrows of those I love pointing away from me. Together forever with Shawn doesn't happen; together lasts not quite three years.

When Shawn breaks up with me, he is gentle and explains that he loves me and cares about me, but just is not *in* love with me anymore. He parts with us remaining friends, but he no longer wants to ride the emotional rollercoaster that comes with dating me. I have no choice in the matter, neither in the break-up nor in staying strapped on the coaster. I don't know how to get the undulating beast of the rollercoaster to stop, and the only way to exit the coaster ride is to jump off of it.

Ride or jump? Ride or jump? In my mind, only a fine line exists between staying on the roller coaster and feeling like I want to die and jumping off and actually dying. In the past, I always thought if I could just hang on, the ride would slow down and eventually end, but it had been going on for so long that I gave up hope that the rollercoaster would ever stop.

I am not afraid to die, thanks to Great-Grandma—at this point, the gift she gave me of no longer fearing death has no advantage. I am more afraid of staying alive in my current forever state of hell-on-earth. My suicidal ideology shifts into seeing death as a sweet release from my torment—a torment that cannot be relieved any other way. I don't want to hurt anyone else; I just want the pain to cease. My mind's torture is excruciating, unignorable, and thorough. Besides, I believe the world and everyone in it is better off without me. I see my suffering state as a permanent one, which requires a permanent solution.

My change in thinking—from passively wanting to die to actively plotting my suicide—may be the result of something as simple as a medication change. Prozac is the new psychiatric drug of choice for treating depression while I'm in college. Eighteen years into the future, the Prozac label contains the FDA black box warning that there is a risk of exacerbating suicidal symptoms—and even of acting on them—at the onset of taking this specific prescription for people in my age group at that time. I only take the pills as prescribed for a month before deciding to end my suffering the only plausible way I know, by killing myself.

At the age of 21, I enact my plan. I swallow my entire bottle of Prozac.

Things are not always as they appear. Shawn, the good friend that he still is, is storing my medication for me in his dorm room at my request, knowing I may be tempted to overdose. When I grab the bottle from

Shawn's dorm room, my medicine looks identical to his prescription bottle of acne medication. What really happens, in my muddled and haphazard state, is that I down his entire bottle of tetracycline. I don't realize this error in the moment. Pills swallowed, I collapse to the floor in a fit of sobbing, immediately regretting my sin. One of Shawn's roommates sees this scenario unfold and snaps into emergency mode. Somehow, through the blur of my breakdown, I scarcely realize that I, and the empty pill bottle, are scooped up, rushed to the hospital, and thrust into the emergency room, where I am convinced I am about to meet God and be reunited with Great-Grandma.

As I writhe on the paper-covered exam table, curtains drawn and overhead lights blinding me, I squint my eyes closed and pray, not realizing I'm babbling out loud and being overheard. "I see the light! Is this the light I am supposed to go into? I'm so sorry. I didn't mean to do it. Oh, God, please forgive me. I made a terrible mistake. Great-Grandma, I'm coming to meet you. I can't believe I'm going to die."

"You're not going to die." I'm snapped out of my frantic prayer by a loud annoyed male. "You're just going to have a bad stomachache." I start upright and flash open my eyes. "Here, drink this." The doctor gestures to the nurse, who hands me a cup of thick gray liquid. It's chalky, mostly tasteless, and I choke it down, as ordered.

I can't believe my luck! The nurse shows me the empty prescription bottle with Shawn's name on it, and I realize the good fortune of my mishap. I swallowed the wrong pills. I am not going to die! At the age of 21, I get a second chance at life.

I signed myself in to the psychiatric unit to avoid a court-ordered hospital stay. On the psych ward, I am diagnosed as "bipolar type II." New meds. New treatment plan. New psychiatrist. I am told I will need both medication and professional counseling for the rest of my life. I am prepared to make the best of it.

Section III

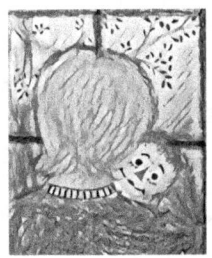

Exposed to the Light

There's something new
   yet something old
   in my closet.
It's behind the clothes
   that mask my mood
   and project "a someone."
It's behind the collectibles
   salvaged from my childhood.
It's a big, dark space
   I'm afraid to enter, a space
   feeling far too familiar
   to be comfortable.
Why haven't I seen it before now?
Surely it's been there all along,
   though invisible to
   denying eyes.
I shoot glances in its direction
   but my eyes quickly dart away.

There's something new
   yet something old
   in my closet

   a dark terrifying void

   I can't bear
   the thought of it
   being there.

CHAPTER 12

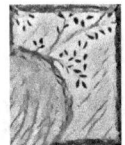

HAPPILY EVER AFTER

Autumn leaves twirled freely in the breeze, swirling with snowflake flurries, as I trekked through my second year on the university campus as a single, eligible coed. One particularly defeating Friday, after classes and before choir, I tried to think: out of all my college friends, who was the one person who could make me laugh just then? Kendal immediately came to mind. He sang bass in our choir and plucked jokes and funny observations out of the air, batting them into casual conversations with perfect aim and timing. He was likable in a light-hearted kind way that made me feel safe and simultaneously amused. We had never done anything one-on-one before, but I decided to invite him to hang out after rehearsal. I really needed to laugh and to not be alone. He was surprised that I singled him out but accepted. We opted for pizza and a video in his dorm room.

Yellowbeard was the movie of choice because Madeline Kahn—whom I adored—was pictured on the box with a cast of swashbuckling Monty Python pirates, and I wanted to see something silly and dumb, just for the fun of it. The movie did not disappoint, neither in its silliness nor in its dumbness. What started out as a casual evening of laughing between friends ended up in an all-night exchange baring of souls. Kendal was easy to talk to, and we developed a genuine fondness for each other in sharing our life stories into the wee hours, past curfew. With our first kiss, the sparks flew, and that clinched it. We were a couple.

Kendal and I bonded: over music—singing and touring with our choir pals; over school spirit—sporting our mascot attire and cheering our teams as raucous fans; over coursework—hunching over textbooks in late-night study sessions; over stick-shifts—me purchasing my first car, him teaching me how to drive a four-on-the-floor, me avoiding busy intersections and hillcrests with stop signs until mastering the clutch. We celebrated holidays with each other's families, road-tripping across the Midwest to eat every dinner, open every gift, kiss every grandparent—a valiant quest with two sets of parents and stepparents between us, making four celebrations per holiday in the space of a three-day weekend, and traversing past miles of cornfield rows in changing seasons of growth.

I already lived off-campus with a roommate and worked to pay for the apartment while finishing my degree. Kendal soon did likewise. After university graduation, the two of us moved into an apartment of our own, no more roommates, just the pair of us and the two cats we adopted. My love knew my history, at least all the history I could recall, and wrapped his arms around all of me, including my psychotherapy sessions, my trips to the pharmacy, my insurance copays, and my mood swings. We were both relieved when my prescription medicine seemed to be working better, and I was released from routine counseling and upgraded to simple monthly medication check-ups. After our four years of dating plus two years of living together, I got the proposal I had been hinting for. Christmas morning, I felt a ring box in my stocking. I cracked open the hinged lid, knowing what was inside. My maternal grandmother's wedding ring (the heirloom my mother bestowed upon Kendal for our engagement) glistened on my finger. Kendal knelt, popped the question and, in my pjs, through my happy tears, of course, I said, "Yes."

Mom remarried in May, wedding her second husband the spring before Kendal and I began dating. I was grateful that my stepdad romanced my mom and doted on her in a way my dad never had. Bigbro and Lilbro had wives of their own, with a baby girl for Lilbro. Most recently, my dad had been "born again" and had married again (wife number three) in early summer just prior to my late summer nuptials with Kendal. All our lives seemed to be heading in better directions. My whole family attended our wedding, and so did Kendal's family, my new in-laws.

So, what happened to my dad's second family? A decade into his second marriage, I got a distraught phone call from Dad.

"I came home from work, and she was just gone! All her stuff and her son's stuff moved out. Not just the clothes, she took all the furniture too. There's barely anything left in the house. Come to find out, she's been having an affair with a guy down the road for months now. She's moved in with him and wants a divorce. I didn't even know she wasn't happy. This is news to me."

"Yeah, it sucks when someone just up and leaves like that, without warning."

"No kidding. I don't know what I'm going to do. I can't afford to live here by myself. I can imagine what the neighbors are saying. This is a small town where everybody knows everyone else's business. I don't know that I can stay here, not if she's staying—and it looks like she is—with that man."

"Uh huh," I can't believe I have to say it. "Now do you have some idea of how we felt when you left?"

Long pause. "Oh… yeah… I guess I did do the exact same thing to your mother, didn't I?… I never thought about it that way…. I didn't think any of you would mind me gone…. Gosh, I never realized. I'm so sorry. I never should have done that, should I?… No, I guess I shouldn't have…. I guess I deserve this don't I?"

"No one deserves to be left, Dad."

"Boy… I'm sure sorry…. This gives me a whole new perspective being on the receiving end."

My dad ends up being better off in the long run. None of the rest of us understood what he saw in wife number two, and we all agreed wife number three was a substantial upgrade.

Kendal and I honeymooned in the Twin Cities (Minneapolis-St. Paul), partly because it was all our budget could afford and partly because we wanted to visit my godmother. Due to agoraphobia, she hadn't left her comfort zone of Minneapolis in years and regretted missing our wedding ceremony.

My memories of the Twin Cities were many, since my childhood family visited there nearly every summer. The five of us, piled in the Rambler station wagon, eagerly spotted the familiar landmarks, indicating we were nearing the big city. First, we would see the towering billboard cutout of The Jolly Green Giant rising from the cornfields as we sped down the highway past the town of the Green Giant/Pillsbury factory. Next, the soundwall barriers lining the interstate rose up on either side, blocking our view of the suburbs while channeling the sounds of traffic whizzing through the lanes. Then, our view of the IDS Tower (the tallest building in Minneapolis), grew on the cityscape horizon through the front windshield, signaling our exit from the freeway onto the inner-city streets. Finally, when we would pull into the driveway and burst out of the car doors, one of us invariably would have to skip the bear hugs, dashing into the house to pee.

Godmother lived in the century-old house where her mother was born, and her sister's family of five lived nearby. Our mix of families, with kids close in age, toured one or more of the local attractions: traversing the Fort Snelling historical army base, visiting exotic animals at the Minnesota Zoo, splashing in the shallow pools at the base of Minnehaha Falls, riding daredevil attractions at the Valleyfair amusement park, searching the best discounts in the Nicolette Shopping District downtown, and peering out the highest point in Minneapolis, the IDS Tower's fifty-fifth-floor observation deck.

I got my love of purple from my love of my Godmother, whose name I treasure as my middle name. Her entire bedroom, from floor to ceiling, was decked out in purples and lavenders, from the plum roses on the wallpaper to the violet shades of shags in the carpet, from the grape chenille bedspread to the periwinkle lace throw pillows, from the magenta hanging ball lamp to the hyacinth striped curtains, from the bluish-red floral bathrobe to the reddish-blue fuzzy slippers. It was my pleasure to get to sleep with her, however many nights we stayed, wrapped snugly in her den of royal purpleness.

Godmother even wore purple—every single day. Her entire wardrobe matched her bedroom palette, with necklaces and scarves, coats and hats, shoes and handbags, shirts and blouses, casual slacks, and Sunday dress—all purple. I wanted to be just like her.

She was a hoot with a lead foot: yelling at drivers to get out of the way; honking at cars—*move it or lose it buddy*; flooring it through the turn—*hang on to your hats;* gassing on the yellows—*that one might have been pink;* screeching to a halt—*whoa Bessy*; and revving at the stop lights until lurching off again—*ready set go*; as she wheeled the careening sedan into a carnival ride. A thrill to survive.

My godmother, an independent feminist, who never married (she had no use for a man and would not be told what to do by anyone) cared for her mother in their rickety home in the inner city. She had a quick wit and an easy, deep belly laugh. She freely shared her opinions, critiquing everyone and everything, accenting her declarations with amusing facial contortions. Her Christian faith was deep and abiding, thus she received the coveted title of Godmother at my and all my siblings' christenings. And she had cats. Lots of them. All over her house. It was a maze of fur and meows, amongst her packrat home decor.

My parents indulged my love of purple with a lavender bedspread, purple carpet, and matching paint and wallpaper, with a few pinks mixed in. Not all my clothes were purple, but my dance leotard always was, and I preferred purple attire to anything else. I stretched the neck of the purple poncho Godmother had knit for me, so I could wear it long after my head struggled to fit through the original hole.

Even though Godmother lived a day's drive away, she kept in touch with holiday cards and birthday greetings throughout the year and always remembered to honor the anniversary of my baptism. The few times she visited us were a treat. Then she could sleep snugly wrapped in my purple haven of royalness.

To this day, purple is my favorite color, and I find it's good for my mental health. Just the sight of it in any tint or shade makes me happier than I would be without it. For me, purple is a visual comfort and a mood lifter, without the side effects of drugs, and a living memorial to my namesake Godmother.

The honeymoon period following Kendal and me saying, "I do," was brief. We got six months of, "for better," before the "for worse," kicked in. And things did get worse. A lot worse. Kendal and I didn't know it would eventually end up better. The foundation of friendship we built a year prior to dating became crucial during the upheaval, while we prayed for better days. Our prayers would go unanswered for many years.

I didn't recognize what was happening at first. After the fact, years later, I was able to look back and see that my buried trauma memories began to surface six months into our marriage. The AM radio now had an FM switch, and it flipped on sporadically, without warning. I retrospectively figured out that these FM interruptions had happened because I finally had a secure home of my own—a safe place in which to remember. My growing up home was not safe, and I felt transient living on my own with roommates in the dorms and apartments. But my marriage felt permanent, our life together, secure.

Bam! A panic attack hit me. This was new to me. The hyperventilation, which had happened during my school-aged years but had ceased when I began taking birth control pills at age 18 and my periods normalized, had numbed me because the rapid, excessive breathing suppressed my emotions.

Panic was hyperventilation's opposite. The halted, limited breathing released painful emotions that overwhelmed me. It happened one night when my husband drove us home after a late evening event. I looked out the passenger side window at the black night sky, watching all the streetlights lining the roadway. I was flushed by a familiar fear—it washed through me—and a thought, "Why does each dot of light in the darkness remind me of light pouring through a keyhole?" A memory flashed in my mind of my childhood bedroom door and the tiny ray of light streaming in from the hallway. A shadow passed over the keyhole, blocking out the light. Fright shook through my body. It took forever to catch my breath. That glimpse of memory knocked me off-kilter, leaving me confused.

Weeks later, *bam!* Another flash. I had gone to bed earlier than my night-owl husband. Alone in our bedroom, I changed into my pajamas, then crawled into bed and turned off the nightstand light. As I settled into sleep, I heard a man's voice, "Turn over and let me feel your bottom." I shrieked. I startled upright. I yanked on the light.

"What's wrong?" Kendal instantly appeared where the man in my imagination should have been.

"He was here! Right here where you're standing. I heard him!" I gasped for breath between sobs.

"He? He who?" Kendal reached out and held me.

I clung to him and cried, "A man! I don't know who. He was here, right next to the bed."

"Well, he's gone now. It's alright, Sweetie, no one's here but me."

I didn't know where the voice came from. I just knew it was real. And it terrified me.

Bam! More panic hit. Kendal had steered us out of a crowded parking lot on a sunny day after a sporting event. We waited in a long line of cars, not moving. A surge of fear coursed through my veins—I felt trapped—I needed to flee, but there was no way out.

Traffic started to crawl. Through the front windshield, Kendal waved in a pickup truck that turned in line in front of us as the vehicles halted to gridlock. The view in front of me was now an empty flatbed. I shielded my eyes and became even more frantic. "Kendal, we have to get out of here, now! I need to get out! We have to go!"

I begged him to make the car move, even though it was impossible. I heard the car's child safety locks click as my fingers grasped the door handle. I froze.

Finally, the traffic started moving again, and we turned onto the main road. Finally, I stopped fidgeting and fretting. If not for Kendal's quick action, I might have jumped out of the car and dashed away. As we drove home, panic turned to tears. What was happening to me?

With these random panic attacks, I developed a startle response. Poor Kendal. There were times when he accidentally frightened me into screaming fits of terror. Each time it happened, I didn't hear him coming and thought I was alone in the house.

One night, I was playing the piano too loudly to hear his approach and was thoroughly absorbed in my music zone, playing and singing with abandon. He opened a door. *Bam!* I screamed bloody murder. My shrieks melted into frightened sobs once I realized I was safe and saw it was only him.

Another day, I was taking a bath, laying my head back and soaking my ears under the water. I didn't answer his calls as he approached from the hallway, so when Kendal reached the bathroom door, he rapped: *knock knock knock. Bam!* Immediate frantic screams—beyond the oh-you-scared-me jump and yelp that happens to others, who then laugh and move on. Way beyond. I let out a death scream.

If panic attacks and startle responses weren't enough to rattle me, I also started having night terrors. My dreaming life had always included the occasional nightmare, where I woke up frightened but was able to shake them off, and roll over and go back to sleep. But these recent nightmares were amplified, intense, vivid, and occurred most every night, ravaging me, exhausting me, haunting me, and extinguishing my ability to function the day after.

The scenarios changed, but the terror didn't: a wild beast chasing after me; a dark figure stalking me; a room imprisoning me; yelling and no one hearing me; seeing a shadow in a doorway; a heavy foot standing on my chest trapping me. The difference between my night terrors and my nightmares was that I couldn't shake the feelings of the terrors once I was awake. I woke up shivering in a cold sweat, crying uncontrollably, and not wanting to go back to sleep, afraid of what new torment awaited me. A pattern emerged with every night terror: the dream would end, and I would be splayed out on the bed, trying to scream. When I finally awoke, I would prop pillows behind me to keep me from rolling onto my back.

I tried journaling, my faithful stress processor and favorite therapy tool from years past. The method—scrawling stream of thought dictation with no effort to censor the content or craft sensible sentences. Putting ink to paper, I allowed the racing thoughts to ramble themselves to extinction. But each stroke of the pen seemed to write me worse instead of better. The words became both a lifeline and a noose, as my inner voice flowed through my pen—a cathartic unleashing of a formerly muted tongue, scribbling:

> He's in my bed again! Make him leave! You never protect me! You let him get away with it! Don't let him touch me! Why didn't you stop him? I hate this Special Game! I hate you!

The message was terrifying to my adult ears, newly hearing it, and to my mature eyes, newly seeing the revelations on the page. I had closed my ears and shut my eyes to that inner voice and vision for so long that I didn't even recognize them as my own, though they had to be mine—they came from the very core of my being and cried out to me with the pain of raw wounds. My adult self dredged up "new" memories—which actually were forgotten memories, blocked memories—shattering all I had ever known into chaos.

It was as if my life were a completed jigsaw puzzle, and someone threw a handful of new pieces at me and said, "Here! Make these fit, too." Before now, I thought I had pressed every tab and slot into its rightful place, the picture finished, nothing missing. Now, upon further scrutiny, I realized the picture was askew. Images aligned improperly. I had mistakenly fit some of the puzzle pieces, forcing them into the wrong places. How had I not noticed this before? More than a mere few areas were misaligned, prongs and crevices haphazardly conjoining, my makeshift collage cobbled with opaque scenes blurring together, obscuring what was absent. Having grown accustomed to the rough edges of my life's jigsaw puzzle, I realized I had been more comfortable keeping the pieces misassembled. Now, I saw the blank spots, the missing pieces, the conflicting sections, and the thought of deconstructing from the beginning overwhelmed me. However, despite the fresh pain, it was unbearable to live this incomplete life.

My hand, possessed by the trauma narrative, inked up page after page of my journal with horrific information. The 29- and 30-year-old me turned into a suspicious defense lawyer, cross-examining the hostile witness about the rabid scribblings. I questioned myself at every turn: "How can this be?" "What are you trying to do to me?" Why are you saying these things?" "You must be crazy!" "Just shut up already!"

As the emotional turbulence of my past and present clashed, apocalyptic natural disasters unleashed within me and around me. I vacillated between childishly spatting with myself and viscerally numbing myself. But I found no shelter in the eye of this storm, as my mind became a cyclone of swirling thoughts, whirling images, twisting emotions, that leveled my memories, destroying my past in its path. The world outside my head became a distant land beyond my reach, a blurred land beyond my focus, a functioning land beyond my comprehension, a happy land well beyond my grasp. Do I still belong to the world? Do I belong anywhere?

I barely navigated daily existence as fragments of memories ambushed me in their varied and intrusive waves. I had to do something. The voices and images were not going away; the invasion was beyond what my daily prescription dose could contain; the Shadow Monster I had learned to tolerate was devolving into something worse. I needed professional help, and I equated this need with abject failure.

I had long since left my college mental health connections behind, and so I had to search for mental health services covered by my insurance. Unfortunately, I avoided calling anyone until I was desperate, and I had to settle for the first available opening with whoever was taking new clients. I just wanted to be well, like an average person who doesn't need therapy. Was that too much to ask? It seemed to be, and I detested my fate of needing help, feeling like an ill child choking on a spoonful of castor oil.

As I entered the office building of this new counselor and proceeded to the waiting room, my feet dragged as my heart raced. I didn't want to be there, talking to another professional about my personal history and current inadequacies in life-coping skills. I submitted my paperwork for the umpteenth time, a process I thought was behind me. Patient history: age 17, diagnosis—major depression; age 21, suicide attempt, diagnosis—manic depression (bi-polar type II). Current reason for seeking therapy: age 31, self-diagnosis—panic attacks, nightmares, sleep disorder, possible depression. I slunk over to the receptionist, handing her the clipboard, my cheeks flushed, my eyes avoiding contact.

"How will you be paying for this today?" asked the frizzy-haired brunette, sporting a medical tag with her name and title, "Receptionist." The plastic name tag dangled at a forty-five-degree angle to the bright red pinstripes of her ruffled-neck blouse. Her lipstick matched the pinstripes perfectly. She pointedly indicated the sign in all caps with her ballpoint, "Payment Due Date Of Service. No Exceptions," and then angled the pen to scratch her head, lips smacking her chewing gum while she awaited my answer.

"My insurance," I placed the laminated card on the counter, "and I'll pay cash for the fifteen-dollar copay."

"That's fine, Hon. I'll ring up the copay now and then verify your policy information while you're in session. Just check back after your session for your receipt." She managed a smile through her gum-gnawing.

"Thank you." I left the card with her and handed over the money. Relieved to leave the counter, I claimed a floral wingback chair among a handful of eye-contact-avoiders (like me) and snagged a magazine. All of us were loafing mindlessly through glossy pages, feigning interest in articles like "8 Steps to a Happier You," or pictures of smiling yachters surrounded by Caribbean islands.

My stomach reminded me with an audible gurgle emanating from where an ulcer had once churned. Trading lunch for a strawberry smoothie today had not had the soothing effect I intended.

At last, I heard my name, "Deborah?" Did they have to say my name so loud? What happened to confidentiality? It was bad enough entrusting my psychiatric history to the gum smacker.

Mr. Therapist looked boyish, around my age, and reminded me of a sheepish big brother. His kind smile would have set me at ease were it not for my mind silently questioning his experience and credentials. After a few pleasantries, I recounted the onset of panic episodes and startle responses. He listened without taking any notes. Then I went on to describe my nightmares. Still, no notes. And relayed my journal entries. No notes. By the end of the session, Mr. Therapist had said little, and he wrote nothing. "I'd like to see you once a week for starters and see how you progress. In the meantime, the staff psychiatrist can give you some anti-anxiety medication to help ease your symptoms. Please bring your journal entries with you to our next session."

I bit my lip while thinking, "Spill my guts to a stranger for an hour and go out into the world like nothing happened. All in a day's work, unless you're the helpee, like I am." I dutifully presented myself to the receptionist, who was again rubbing her scalp with the ballpoint.

"It seems you have a $600 deductible for mental health care, Hon. That means your copay doesn't kick in until you have met the deductible in full. I have your itemized bill minus the fifteen dollars you gave me. Here's your insurance card. That will be one-hundred ten dollars, please."

I stared at her, stunned. I had already met the deductible when seeing my regular physician. Why was my mental health care any different?

"How would you like to pay for that? Cash or personal check?" More gum cracking and pen scratching.

"Ah... ah... check please." It was all I could do to choke back my tears. My eyes filled, blurring my penmanship as I filled out the check, a single teardrop smeared my signature.

"Would you like to reschedule?"

The question echoed in my ears. "Ah... I left my pocket calendar at home. I'll... ah... have to call you," I lied, as I ripped the last remaining check away from the carbon imprint and handed it over.

"Oh, I see you have a prescription note request. That office is down the hallway and around the corner, just before you get to the elevators. It says, 'Walk-In Prescription Clinic' on the door. They do their billing separately. Here's your receipt, Deborah. Have a nice day." Again with the sideways smile, as she pushed the papers and card across the counter.

I grabbed her offerings and stuffed them into my handbag with the empty checkbook and dodged down the hallway. I hurried past the legal drug-pushers, feeling as guilty and conspicuous as a prisoner caught in a searchlight, as fluorescent light glared down on me from above. They'll have figured out I skipped out on my medicine, but I had no means to pay for it now. It seemed an hour's journey to reach the thank-goodness-it-was-empty elevator and to take refuge there as the heavy doors rolled shut.

Gulp-like gasps echoed in the chamber—my attempt to suffocate the erupting sobs. This panic was not from a vortex unknown. It was from the fear of a passerby witnessing my full meltdown. Fortunately, there was no one waiting on the ground floor, and I voiced a frail "thank you" as I ducked past a sportscoated man holding open the outside building door.

Once in the car, the torrent unleashed. Gut-wrenching waves of desperate cries erupted, "I can't afford to be sick!" I angrily wept, "I can't afford to get help! Why? Why? Why?" The third pound of my fists on the steering wheel set off the horn, startling me with an abrupt scream. Then silence. All I could hear was my labored breathing. My skin tingling, my hair rising, like a rabbit on alert after fleeing to safety. Spent and numb, I turned the key, revved the engine, and steered toward home in an autopilot trance.

What was worse? The stress of being mentally ill, the stress of seeking help, or the stress of paying for treatment? All three contributed to my downward spiral as I stepped past my threshold into the apartment. I was inconsolable, but Kendal reassured me that we had good credit, and he would simply deposit a credit card check into our bank account so my check for today's appointment wouldn't bounce. It would be okay for me to call the receptionist to schedule follow-up appointments tomorrow, as well as return to the clinic pharmacy to fill the new anti-anxiety prescription.

Would relying on credit card debt leave us bankrupt? Kendal said we would manage. I was as grateful to Kendal for his support as I was aware of our imbalanced alliance—me making emotional messes, him cleaning them up, me adding expenses to our household, him trying to pay the bills, me stretched beyond my limits, him holding us faithfully together.

Mr. Therapist, still hands-free, grasped neither pen nor paper for any of my visits. I brought my journal entries to each session as requested. This time, I relayed to the therapist the occasion the past summer when my dad was planning to visit me for the first time since walking me down the aisle on my wedding day.

"I was extremely anxious about this upcoming visit with my dad, but I don't know why. It was the first time I recall since my parents' divorce that Dad was coming specifically to see me, in my own home, instead of me meeting him at his mother's house—my grandma's house back in my hometown. I couldn't bring myself to tell my dad I didn't want him to come. I had no tangible explanation to give him, just a feeling of not wanting him here. What's that about? Kendal had to call my dad and explain that this wasn't a good time for him to visit, that I was having some problems with past issues that involved him, even though I couldn't pinpoint what they were."

I began to share, reading aloud to Mr. Therapist from a long journal entry that ended with:

> "This suit fits like my birthday suit, but you choose to confuse the two, undressing me with icy precision and not just with your eyes. I hear a man's voice, 'Let me help you with your buttons and your zipper.' I have no idea what I am writing. I only know I'm breathing fast and nervous to think my brain would invent such things while my loins tingle. The guilt is horrible. What am I writing? This pen seems beyond my control at times, as things were then out of my control...
> I couldn't control... he lost control... there's no

control left. Why are we alone? Where is everyone else? Are we supposed to be quiet? There's no lock on the door. It's broad daylight for Chrissake! Sun is shining through the second story window, but I am facing away. I can see the whole room, my childhood bedroom, even behind him. I don't want to look at his face. I don't want to see his hands on my shirt buttons and zipper either. Who is this man with me? Who is this girl in this room, a childhood's bedroom with a father figure? Why would someone look at someone so young in that way with those eyes? I guess it's the way it's supposed to be. But who is this girl? I've only had night, dark and shadow images before, but it's broad daylight. It's the same bed against the opposite wall. It's the same door with the same keyhole. What am I saying? I just don't know. Do I wish these images upon me and myself? Why would I want to do that? Why would I want to invent such a horribly painful memory that is incomplete, but still sends me screaming into oblivion? Do I have such a wild imagination that my nervous system responses mirror the storyline? I'm not even sure if I should write in pen because I can't erase. I can't take back anything I remember once it's in my head and on paper. The memories are locked away. I must find and turn the key. An honest look is my only mission. I'm looking for answers, not hyped-up opinions of 'maybes.' I deserve to heal. The infection must be removed by reopening a wound. This wound is not self-inflicted, and the party responsible must be identified without a doubt for me to be satisfied. It's the only assurance of an accurate antidote. The ability to put a face with the crime will either free or convict my father. My father is on trial in my own mind. There is just not enough evidence to verdict him guilty at this time. There's a motive, opportunity and much suspicion, but no eyewitness. I don't want to accuse an innocent man. I want to deal with facts and reality. I need more facts. The person had a face. Surely if I can remember the unimportant details, I can recall a simple face of shame that has somewhere burned my memory."

I paused as I finished reading, visibly shaken. "That's it. I'm still stuck. I can't see his face. I don't know for certain who abused me." The emotions that stirred from reading the words had no resting place.

Mr. Therapist's mouth gaped into astonished disbelief, and asked, "You have no idea who your abuser is?"

"No," I responded, "I told you, I can't see his face."

"You mentioned eyes, those eyes looking at you. Whose eyes are they?"

"I don't know. It's just the eyes I see, and then they fade away."

His frustration with me unleashed into an accusatory tirade, his mild demeanor shifting into a fierce inquisition. "Do you really have to see his face to know who it is? My God! How can you not know when it is all right in front of you, written in black and white, by your own hand? How can you not hear it when you read it out loud? How can you not see it when the clues are everywhere? I know who it is! You don't have to tell me!" He reined himself in a bit, now looking defeated and muttering, "No, you have to wait and see it for yourself. I can't tell you who it is, but I know, and he doesn't deserve the benefit of the doubt." Mr. Therapist might as well have slapped me across the face. I flushed with righteous indignation at his inappropriate breach of ethics. Of course, I knew he thought it was my dad, he doesn't have to say it. I wanted him to be wrong. That's the last face I wanted to see in my memories. I wanted the blur to clear and reveal somebody else, anybody else—but please—not Dad.

Both shaken and furious, I terminated the session by exiting prematurely, fleeing his office, thinking, "I'm done! I'm outta here! Time for a new therapist." I never wanted to set foot in this clinic again. Thankfully, my copay had kicked in, so I marched past the reception desk without stopping. I hurried down the hall, half thinking, half muttering, "I'm definitely seeking out a female counselor to talk to from here on out, and someone that specializes in sexual abuse. I cannot handle any more male posturing. This time, I am doing my research, and not subjecting my mental health to the first available opening." I needed experienced help for the long haul.

My new psychotherapist, Ms. Lynn, exuded genuine kindness and compassion, and I liked her right away. At our first visit, I relayed my most recent Mr. Therapist experience. She offered me the option of filing a complaint. Already battling enough internally, I didn't have the energy for an external fight. I just wanted to move on, and so we did.

We started with hypnotherapy. It was not initiated to retrieve my memories, but to help cope once my memories surfaced on their own, processing my known trauma into healthy releases. I had the best luck with guided imagery. These hypnotic sessions encouraged me to create a safe place within myself to rest and heal.

I pictured a grassy meadow of wildflowers, tucked into a hillside. Here, I sat back as my full-bodied adult self was enfolded in Great-Grandma's lap. Together we leaned against a sturdy oak, shaded by its canopy. Below us we gazed at the glistening surface of an oval pond, with a stream for a tail that wound and reached past a sandy shore, into cascading ocean waves. Sea breezes stirred from below, casting a sweet floral fragrance, lightly salted. Blue sky. Warm sun. Chirping birds. Perfumed flowers. With just us and nature, all was right with the world, and in this mutual, interior moment, I was held, beyond words, feeling safe, knowing love.

Early in our sessions together, and with my further journaling, my worst fear materialized. The blurred face shifted into clear focus and left no question, no mystery, no doubt.

I saw Dad—Dad's face, Dad's eyes, Dad's smirk, Dad's deeds. My dad molested me, and the memories of the Special Game he instigated came flooding back, showing how it started, recalling how it repeated, revealing how it escalated, and finally knowing how it ended. As a child experiencing his incest, I found it novel, confusing, uncomfortable, annoying, disquieting, invasive, and finally terrifying. As an adult newly remembering his incest, it disgusted me, it embarrassed me, it pained me, it violated me, it disillusioned, infuriated, and outraged me—it was gut-wrenchingly awful in every possible way.

Ms. Lynn and I strategized several scenarios for confronting him, first, and then my mom. Since there is no win-win scenario possible when calling out a perpetrator and an accomplice, I decided on the best approach for me—writing a letter to my dad, and then placing a phone call to my mom.

My letter to Dad was a brief, handwritten note, scribbled inside a blank card, and dropped in the mail:

> Dad,
>
> You'll be happy to know that my incest therapy is going well. Your "special game" has cost me years of my life and much anguish. I'm sure you remember far better than I. Don't bother denying it because we both know it's true. I wish to have no further contact with you.
>
> DK

I let Bigbro know about the note with a phone call. I kept him in the loop, even though he didn't know what to think when I told him my incest memories. I figured he would be the first one Dad would call upon receiving my note, and I didn't want Bigbro to be blindsided.

It turns out, confronting mom was a bit easier, as she happened to call me. I wrote this journal entry after our conversation:

> Mom just called. The gist is I told her my memories and about the note I wrote to Dad. She said

it seemed out of character for him and admitted she didn't know what to say. She agreed I had no reason to lie, and said she'd have to think about it, but at the moment she had no suspicious memories and did not remember the "special game" argument with me or Dad. She said she understood why I didn't want to talk to Dad, but offered no further support by asking the protective motherly questions. In between the above thoughts, she would comment on her environment. "I'm cleaning the lime off the sink handle and now I can't get it to shut off." "Oh, here comes your aunt. She must be off work," pausing to have a side conversation with Auntie. Meanwhile, I just listen. For what? I'm not sure. Maybe a little more concern, maybe a little more outrage that her baby's been harmed, some afterthought of protection would be nice. But that's not Mom. At least she didn't stick up for him, even if she didn't stick up for me either. As far as I know, she's still on my side.

Bigbro called to tell me that Dad denied everything, and our dad thinks I am the victim of some adverse psychotherapy technique or a medication side-effect. Dad said he will respect my wishes and not contact me and, any forced encounters (family weddings or funerals), he'll handle with mutual, polite avoidance.

My memories began and ended with me. No one involved corroborated the abuse I endured—not my mom, not my dad. Then and now, I was alone with my pain.

If only Raggedy Ann could talk. She was there. She knew and could verify every damnable encounter. But no matter how I wished it, *Toy Story* was just a movie, and Raggedy Ann posed silent with her knowing smile.

There once was a four-year-old girl with blonde wisps of hair and large darkest brown eyes who was handed a grenade by her father. The father said this was a special gift, so special that no one else could know about it. She was warned not to pull the pin, by telling, or the special gift would be ruined forever.

The girl felt extra special to be given such a fascinating gift. But it was very hard to find a safe hiding place where no one would find it. She decided to swallow it whole, which she did. After a while, she forgot she'd ever been given the grenade. Until one day, years later, when the little girl was now a woman, she had a horrible stomachache. It had been noticeable for years, but no medicine could cure it. The woman had the idea to reach down her throat for an object for reasons unknown. Sure enough, she found the grenade and pulled it out and stared at it. Her adult eyes could now see what her child eyes did not. She stared at it until the memories of Daddy's special gift, given only to her, returned.

The woman no longer wanted the grenade but knew there was no safe place to hide it, and the only way to get rid of it was to pull the pin and let it detonate. So, she ignored her childhood father's warning, and told the secret. She pulled and threw.

The grenade exploded, as she knew it would.

The aftermath of this explosion is what the rest of my therapy dealt with, and it resembled a wasteland within me.

*O*nce she forgot to remember,
then she remembered she forgot.

Chapter 13

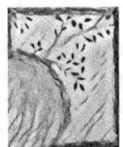

Forgetting to Remember

Why, in my early 30s, was I blindsided by buried memories? It made logical sense why I buried them in the first place. The childhood incest was initially too devastating to bear and later too heinous to conjure. The teenage rape too violating to name, too destructive to claim.

My young survival depended on preserving a semblance of normalcy over chaos, covering the trauma—forgetting. Forgetting in order to survive.

How ironic that my adult survival depended on revealing the underlying chaos, exposing the trauma—remembering. Remembering in order to Survive. (This may explain why my parents don't remember. The opposite holds true for them. Their adult survival still depends on forgetting. In remembering, they have nothing to gain and everything to lose.)

My forgotten trauma blindsided me because, for the first time in my life, I had a safe place to remember. But, even within this safe place, the process of remembering felt fatal.

How can I explain to you, Dear Reader, what it was like? No single metaphor is adequate, and no simple narrative can begin to encompass the complexities I experienced: the polarized thoughts of disparate memories, the conflicting emotions of alternate realities, the layers of trauma inside the past victims (each age, each incident requiring its own healing). They collectively compounded, bewildering the present-day me. Images of natural disasters, of floods and earthquakes, of volcanos and tornadoes occur simultaneously and out of nowhere, as do stampedes of wild horses—parts of myself fleeing to safety—and the adult me burrowing to avoid the bombardment.

Attempting to layer the metaphors and link them might help you experience the chaos of the healing path I experienced, a path not straight from point A to point B but a messy scribble of jagged lines and swirling smudges that crisscross and overlap, with no clear beginning, middle, or end. I invite you into my world.

Think back to Earth Science class in elementary school and picture the 3-D globe. Imagine the space within my abdomen filled with a miniature earth, a living, breathing planet, and my subconscious is everything beneath the Earth's surface. The Earth's inner core and deepest layer (an iron ball) holds the trauma; the core is centered in the unhealed emotions of the outer core (metal lava). The next layer, called the lower mantle, has trapped the 3-4-5-6-7-year-old victims of this trauma. The adjacent upper mantle layer traps the 13-year-old victim.

Guarding the continental crust, the Shadow Monster tries to keep the victims, their emotions, and their traumas, layered beneath the surface, but weird sensations emerge and swirl in the oceanic crust, creating the currents of unexplained symptoms (hyperventilation, migraines, depression, mania) felt in the conscious me that resides on the earth's surface. During childhood and beyond, the outer world was not safe enough to expose the world I held within, so I had to keep it hidden, even from myself.

Later, when Kendal's steadfast love sturdied me, when our bond proved firm with time, when we solidified our devotion through marriage vows, the security I felt in our union jolted tectonic plates, creating a fault line between the crumbling past and the rising future, upheaving a new foundation. This sacred ground of our love was the safe place I had always longed for but had never known. However, the same earthquake that allowed the new foundation to emerge also cracked open a gorge, reaching to the depths of the buried captives, freeing them.

My abused inner child and inner teenager twins, wise enough to hide when the outer world wasn't safe, were also savvy enough to recognize this new bedrock would provide the firm footing required for the strenuous healing to come. The captives, along with their trauma memories and raw emotions, rushed forward like wild horses, thundering a stampede of truths, unearthing the terrain of my life. My wounded captives, who had found a new home with Kendal, fled their underground prison and were galloping to safety, a place where they could be seen, heard, held, and healed.

However, the kicked-up dust felt anything but safe to the adult me, and I didn't know if I would survive a dust storm of endless debris.

After a honeymoon grace period of six months, Post-traumatic Stress Disorder (PTSD) symptoms trampled our wedded bliss. It took me six months to realize I'd forgotten some sort of childhood trauma. It took me another six months to understand that the trauma was me being molested as a child, and over six more months to show me the perpetrator was my father. With some more time and memory fragments, I recognized that my mom knew about the sexual abuse. I acknowledged my family wasn't perfect, and neither was my childhood growing up. Whose is?

But this new, disjointed information didn't fit with all the things I'd always known. And then, just when I thought I had remembered every horrible thing I had buried in my past, the rape memories with the three guys in a truck came hurtling back. More time elapsed. There was too much chaos to integrate. Trauma memories swirling within me and around me blocked my vision. I was stuck, paralyzed, unable to escape. My journal tells more:

> I wake, but not from the daymare. It doesn't go away, this daymare of my reality. And I don't want it. I want to wake without this immediate abuse realization. Why must it relentlessly torment me so? Why can I not honor it 1 hour a day instead of 24? It is always there. Maybe this is all my life has ever been and all it will ever be. I want some semblance of a normal life. Everyone else seems

to have it. I may as well have died. Death would be more gracious than this shell of a life. Nothing has changed but me. It feels like eternal damnation among the living. Why am I deserving of such torture? Why me? It's like a neon flashing light in my head strobing, "Incest! Incest! Incest!" There is no off switch. It's too big to cover up, it's too bright to block out, it's too insistent to ignore.

With my memories revealed, my captive twins freed, the Shadow Monster's reason to exist vanished, and its presence disappeared, the banished pain was left unprotected, raw, and seething. I amazed myself at how smoothly I conducted the business of work and public life for a few years, while thundering hooves stampeded across a volcanic field. I struggled to prevent lava inside me from erupting. No one saw the smoldering person beneath the facade, teetering on the rims of the volcanos, one trip-step away from sacrificing herself to the gods. They only saw my agility as, behind the smokescreen, I scaled rocky terrain, balanced at dizzying heights, and forged my inner fires into my work responsibilities. But work exhausted me, and I had nothing left over for myself or for Kendal when I collapsed at home. This public illusion gradually melted as tremors rumbled, molten rock flared, and the river of fire engulfed my life, making engaging in the world—even for as little as an hour at a time—impossible.

I shielded myself from the lava spill, digging in at home, hiding from commitments, delving downward into depression. My freshly scalded wounds left me feeling frail, vulnerable, exposed, and unprotected. It became arduous to leave the house, so I cowered, shades drawn, covered in blankets, burrowed into the couch, staring at whatever happened to flit across the TV screen. When I did go out, I was afraid others could see the tortured soul I desperately tried to conceal, and I feared my inner pain and panic would seep into my public persona.

Triggers appeared at every turn: in the park, a father pushed his daughter on a swing, and my eyes spilled tears; two teen girls whizzed by on ten-speed bikes, and I cringed from head to toe; a family in the grocery store pushed a little girl in a shopping cart, and I lamented she might be being abused. These types of scenes loomed over me, both as reminders of how things should have been and as reminders of how things never should have been.

Hiding from commitments included hiding from work. Since graduation, I had earned my living from the same company as I had throughout college. In my entry-level staff position, I directly cared for children and adults diagnosed with developmental disabilities, assisting them in living as independently as possible. Upon graduation, I was promoted to middle management, coordinating services for my clients by overseeing staff, reporting to caseworkers, and communicating with guardians, job-site supervisors, activity directors, and medical care professionals.

While simultaneously processing my own memories, work proved too much for me. Personally, a dust storm continued to swirl up from the memories stampeding over the emotional caldera terrain.

Professionally, work churned a thunderstorm over the plateau, and a torrential downpour gully washed a floodplain. I watched myself going under, drowning in paperwork, drowning in meetings, drowning in the present, drowning in trauma, drowning in the past. I ended up exhausting all my paid sick leave, forced to request a leave of absence through FMLA, the Family Medical Leave Act. This three-months' leave without pay increased financial hardship; our credit card debt grew, but, unable to function in my job, it was my sole option.

Once I filed and signed paperwork for my leave, it seemed the best way to quell any office rumors was to come clean. I spilled my living nightmare of recovering trauma memories to my job cohorts. My supportive colleagues generously donated vacation days to my leave, assuming I would return to work with them again afterward. That eventuality did not happen. I was unaware of how much stress my job entailed until I stopped doing it. I performed it well enough, and it paid the bills, so I never questioned whether or not it was good for me.

This first phase of remembering my buried past was disorienting and exhausting, especially for me, but vicariously for Kendal. He should have had his own counselor to support him in my struggle, but the thought never occurred to us. I don't know how he managed the weight of my reliance on him, the emotional dependence, the debt-juggling amongst zero-percent interest credit cards, the worrying about me being left home alone while he worked, the lack of equal partnership.

Kendal and Ms. Lynn were my lifelines. At least I had no work responsibilities right now; there was nothing I had to do, no one I had to care for, nowhere I had to be, other than in the counseling office twice a week. The chain-reaction consequence of speaking the truth was like tipping the first in a long line of dominoes. I always fell first, and then watched as people close to me—people whom I loved dearly—were tipped over, falling one by one, as they heard my latest news, knocked over by one unbelievable story after another. My journal entry explains how it was for me.

> I'm stuck. I cannot have a real relationship with anyone in the family who doesn't know. But anyone I tell, if they don't outright deny it, sits on the "I can't/don't want to believe it" fence. Do I have a family? Then? Now? Do I have a family? I'm afraid that I don't. I can't pretend around people that don't know about the incest, and I can't pretend around people who do know and don't believe me. They can't pretend to believe in me and still have doubts about my truth. I'm too overwhelmed by the hurt and the loss on so many levels. The memories themselves are too much. The disillusion of my family history is too much. The changing family relationships now are too much. The impact this has had on my personal and professional life is too much.
>
> They say, "The truth shall set you free."
> My truth has imprisoned me, then and now.
>
> Trying to deal, additionally, with family denial and uncertainty, clouds my healing. It's too confusing and frustrating just to see my truth, let alone

trying to persuade others to see it and honor it. It drains all of my energy to be the go-between between myself and family members. I need to be myself right now, all by myself. Maybe later, I can be a daughter and a sister and a granddaughter, too, but only to those who can honor me by honoring my truth. The pretending stops here with me. I know I'm the one who has to stop it.

When I told Ms. Lynn that I felt all alone in the world and felt like nobody understood what I was going through, she just happened to be facilitating the start of another round of group therapy for sexual assault survivors. I both did and didn't want to join. It was a 90-minute meeting once a week on Monday evenings.

The first session, I, along with seven other participants and two leaders, fidgeted in a circle of ten chairs, with only an open floor between us. I sized up my peer group, surprised at how normal these women all appeared, noting not one of them looked like the victim of a horrific sex crime. Maybe I didn't either. Some of the group members knew each other, as the configuration re-formed every eight weeks, with the option to drop out, graduate, or recommit to the next eight sessions, with new members able to join at that time. There were two other new members besides me. The point was to share my story, out loud, with like-traumatized sympathetic people. It was a group I didn't want to be qualified for. None of us did. Yet here we were.

It helped me to hear others' stories throughout our meetings, though it was also hard to witness so much pain. I found myself grateful and guilty that both my incest and rape stories were not the worst tales shared. At least my dad had stopped molesting me. At least my rapists were strangers, and I never had to continue to interact with them. At least I had a supportive husband that honored my need for a break from sex and did not leave me because I wouldn't "put out." At least some of my family believed me and did not disown me. I was not alone. The meetings were a mixture of comfort (to have comrades in my battle to heal) and discomfort (that our numbers were so great). This was where I first heard the one in four statistic. One in four? A chill ran through me when I realized how many children like us had already been sexually abused or would be before the age of 18.

A pretty, married mother of two young boys, graduated when the eight weeks were done. I wanted to be her, able to smile and laugh, to be ahead of the father-daughter incest that ailed her teenage years, ready to go out into the world with renewed energy, confidence, and hope. I was not her. Not yet. Maybe someday.

For our first apartment, my husband and I purchased an upright piano I found advertised for $50 in the classified ads. Playing my old compositions was still a balm for me. I'd leave the world behind temporarily, between the PTSD symptoms and waves of remembering. In my early thirties, when I finally pooled together all of the trauma memories, I began composing again, but the creative process was different. My melodies surged, urgent and pressing. New music came pouring through me. New lyrics came from somewhere and attached themselves to those notes. Whether I wanted to or not, I began to process my pain through songwriting. Or maybe I should say that creativity poured through me, like a tidal wave of feverish obsession, or a waterfall of crazed possession, with me as a mere conduit for the songs being written by the waters flooding through me.

Back in college I wrote "Four Walls" and didn't fully understand what it was about. I knowingly felt like depression was my cage, holding both the Shadow Monster and me, so I could never escape. Each time I sang the song, the first line and a later phrase I wrote never made sense to me.

I'm hiding in these four walls that are myself that I built to keep them out... how can I construct a cage so cruel, almost as bad as what they did to me....

Who were *them* and *they*? *Them* and *they* turned out to be my rapists. When I wrote it, I could feel the four walls, even though I didn't have conscious access to the seven-year-old or the thirteen-year-old trapped within them. It turned out that the song was about so much more. My thirteen-year-old captive must have written both the music and the lyrics back then.

New songs were birthed through me. The former captives could, by claiming the truth, finally grow and develop and mature through music. They took over my grown fingers playing on the keys and my adult voice singing their lyrics. Each song gave me a novel womb to nurture my pain and a newborn cry to express it. The grief was pushed out of me onto the page, into the keys, and released through my vibrato. As I played, I could barely see through the tears or sing through the crackles in my throat. I had no choice in the matter, as both the birthing mother and the midwife. The songs growing inside had to emerge, had to be swaddled upon arrival, handled with care, and tended as any newborn would be.

My songs breathed new life through my guitar during this composition-download period, as well. The arpeggio composition from eighth grade—that I'd always hummed the tune to—now had words. The acoustic lullaby became "Waiting for Rain," the lyrics about wanting to cry, needing to cry, and finally being able to. I knew the wounded thirteen-year-old in me wrote this song, too—the music then, and the words now. The lasting soothing melody beckoned new meaning.

*My porcupine tongue
has yet to injure.
My dagger eyes
are never thrown.
My clenched fists
are always open.
My fire breath
is never burned.*

*I won't surrender
unused weapons.*

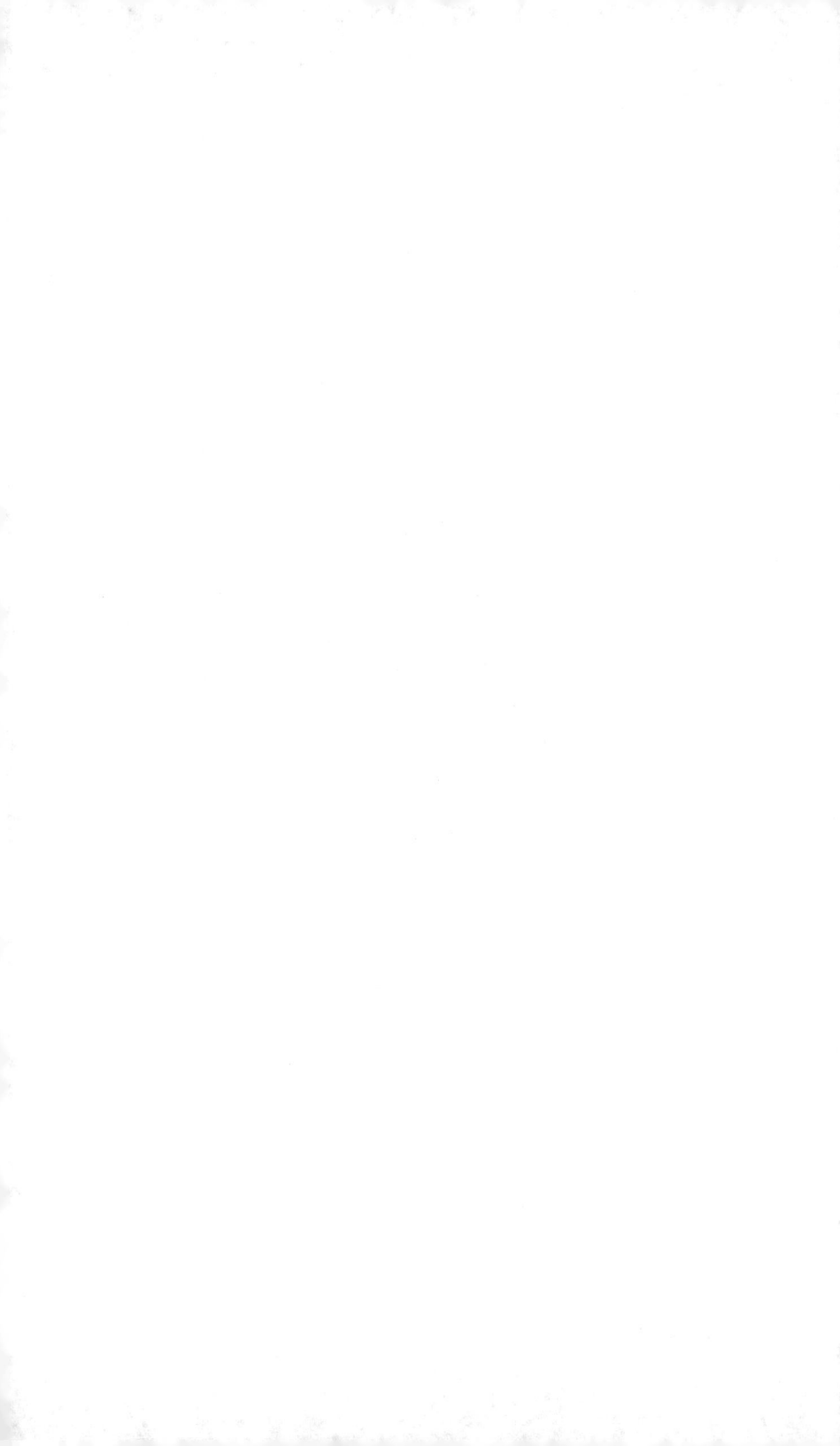

CHAPTER 14

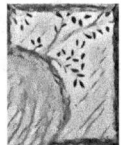

ANGER: MY SUPERPOWER

I was well-versed in both tapping into and expressing the sadness and grief of my healing process. These permissible emotions from my growing-up years, though distressful, felt safe to release. Anger, however, was a different tune. I felt it. I bottled it. I ate it. Sometimes it blew up without warning. Sometimes I blew up without warning. Anger was not safe. I was afraid of it, and afraid I was like my dad.

Prior to his departure, Dad was dependable, but unpredictable. With him as the provider, my family always had a nice home, plenty to eat, good medical care, and, without fail, he attended every recital, ball game, musical performance, and parent-teacher conference for his children, along with Mom and assorted grandparents. When it came to Dad's temper, however, I recoiled.

During my turbulent teens that seemed overly angsty even to me, my signature anger move was to slam a door. After I was done yelling about whatever it was that set me off, the door slam was a satisfying exclamation point that signaled the end of my tirade. I banged my bedroom door as I retreated inside to sulk, or clattered the back door as I exited the house in a huff. My parents were tired of my theatrics and disapproved of my chosen emphasis, and I heard them shout after me as I marched away, "Don't slam the door!" *Slam!* Every time.

Then, one mealtime, in my mid-teens, I slammed my last door. The scene was an evening supper—all five of us clinking utensils and slurping two-percent milk.

"Pass the fried chicken, please," I eyed the drumstick and nabbed it with the tongs. "So, there's this party all the band kids are going to and I want to go—please, pass the mashed potatoes." I dabbed a heaping spoonful onto my plate.

"Where's it at?" Mom asked.

"It's at Billy Turner's house, he's one of the drummers. He lives on Galvin Street near the high school."

"Billy Turner's a dweeb," Lilbro said grinning.

"No, he's not. You don't even know him. He's a nice boy and so is his family."

"I know Billy. He's a decent kid," Bigbro said.

"Anyone who invites you to a party is a dweeb," Lilbro laughed, and we exchanged rolled-eye grimaces.

"Anyway," I continued, "all the band kids are going, and it's Friday night at his house after the football game. Lenee said I can catch a ride with her. Her sister's driving. Can I go?" I hoped they would say yes. *Please* say yes.

"Will Billy's parents be home?" Mom asked.

The dreaded question I was hoping to avoid. "No, they're out of town, but they know about the party and told him he could have it. His 20-year-old sister is staying with him and she'll be the chaperone."

Dad said, "You know the rules: no parents, no party."

"But Dad, his parents know about it and there will be an adult there."

"A sister is not a parent," Dad reminded me.

Bigbro chimed in, "I know Billy's sister. Becky, right? She won't let them get into any trouble."

"That's right. Becky is very responsible and is on a full-ride scholarship," I added, and gave Bigbro an approving nod.

"She's still not a parent," Dad wouldn't budge.

"But Lenee's parents are letting her go and they know Billy's parents won't be there. They know Becky and trust her." I held out hope, as he and I both knew Lenee's parents ran a stricter household than ours.

Dad emphasized, "Well, I don't know Becky or Billy's parents, but I know the parents won't be there so there is no party."

"But there is a party, and everyone is going to be there," I whined.

"Everyone except you. I can't let you go," he insisted.

"Yes, you can! You can totally let me go! You just don't want to! This is so unfair! I have to miss out on the best party of the year just because the parents, who know about the party and okayed the party and happened to appoint a chaperone to the party, won't be there. We're just a bunch of band kids. Nothing's going to happen," my last plea unraveled.

"You're right. Nothing is going to happen because you won't be there." He kept eating his chicken.

"I can't believe this! You're really not letting me go? Everyone else can go but I can't?" I pounded my fists, rising from the table, stomping to the back door, already ajar. "You're ruining my life on purpose just because you can! Because of some stupid rule you made up. I hate you!" I took one more step, turned and with all my strength slammed the door shut behind me. *Bang!*

I wasn't two steps into my stride when, in one swift motion, the door flew open, my dad plucked me up around the waist, hoisted me off my feet, yanked me back into the house, slammed the door himself, and hurled me backward midair, smack into the door, yelling, "I've told you for the last time to stop slamming doors!"

My spine crashed against the solid wood, knocking the wind out of me. Doubled over, I struggled to breathe.

"Stop it! Just stop it!" Mom shouted and came to shield me.

"You can't throw her around like that!" Bigbro yelled and checked on me, "Are you okay?" as I gasped for breath.

Lilbro froze in his chair, staring at us.

Dad, still in a huff, stomped down the basement stairs and back up, white knuckles gripping the toolbox in one hand, then marched down the hallway toward my bedroom. "You like slamming doors? Well you're going to have one less door to slam!" I heard dad hammering the linchpins free from hinges, creaking the wood out of the frame and saw him haul my bedroom door down the basement stairs. I was gobsmacked! How could a teenage girl not have a door to her bedroom?

When I could breathe again, and after the frozen tension lessened to an icy chill, and while the refrigerator stored the half-eaten meal in Tupperware containers, and as the rest of my family retreated to the couch to watch *Laverne & Shirley,* I gaped at the gaping hole in the door frame that exposed my former privacy for all to see. I was shocked that Mom liked the idea, and my brothers both thought the bare opening was hilarious.

"How am I supposed to get dressed or change my clothes?" I fretted.

"You can take your clothes and change in the bathroom," Mom suggested.

I couldn't believe she was going to go along with this. Humiliated, which I guess was the point, but also slightly terrified, I felt like a zoo animal, with everyone able to view anything and everything I used to do behind the privacy of my formerly closed door. My teen sanctuary was ripped away. I felt violated.

My punishment for slamming the doors seemed out of proportion to me but appropriate to everyone else. What was Dad's punishment for slamming me? Nothing. He always got away with being angry. Usually my dad just stomped around and yelled like me. This was the first and last time he flung me, and he hadn't raised a hand to me since I turned too old for childhood spankings. My punishment as an adolescent had switched to docking my allowance, taking away my TV privileges, or grounding me. Now this.

"When am I getting my door back?" I asked, hoping it was a joke and Dad would put the door back in place before bedtime. I always slept with the door closed.

"When you've learned your lesson," he said.

This was no joke. Dad did not relent. Mom failed to come to my defense. I scrambled for a makeshift solution and fastened a sheet to the frame to drape where the door used to be. It was better than nothing, but it felt insecure. There was no longer a lock, not without a door. Nothing prevented anyone from waltzing right in any time they wanted to. It was not that I consciously thought anyone would, it just unnerved me knowing that they could, that I could not stop them. Even if my control over my personal space had been an illusion, it had vanished now. The Shadow Monster grumbled. I froze in fear—a fear from long ago that I couldn't name but felt eerily familiar—and a current fear of keeping the Shadow Monster's existence hidden from the outer world, my family members included. A stunned me inwardly numbed.

How long was my bedroom door missing? More than a month and less than a year. Long enough that the new family joke at my expense—whenever I got mad—was, "Deborah, go slam your sheet!" My dad said it. Bigbro said it. Lilbro said it. Even my mom said it. A lot and often. When they all reminisce about my sheet era, it's still funny to them nearly 40 years after the fact. It was never funny to me, and I don't imagine it ever will be.

In my next session with Ms. Lynn, she assured me there were safe ways to express my anger. I couldn't imagine what that would look like. "A healthy anger release is a planned strategy during which time the felt anger is exhausted and no one gets hurt," she explained. I was still lost. She suggested I start by writing angry letters to people who have hurt me, letters that I would never intend to send. I would have the option in my sessions to read them to her or not.

A tirade of swear words and foul names blew out of my pen like fire, singeing the pages, each word a branding scar of my rage. The reopened memory door fanned the smoldering coals from decades of concealed pain into flames of outrage. I torched my abusers, scorching Dad's excuses, searing Mom's blame, charring the rapists' defenses, blazing their sins. Three fiery letters. Three raging bonfires. Three piles of perpetrators' ashes. A trifecta of arson revenge.

I exhaled words of fire, like dragon breath, in three consecutive psychotherapy sessions, smoking out first my pedophile dad, then my complicit mom, and last the despoiler rapists. Scribbling out my anger empowered me; orating my anger emboldened me; decimating the anger-filled pages freed me.

When anger left my body, it transferred to the letters. There, trapped within the words on the page, my anger had simply found a new home. Crumpling the unsent correspondence and tossing it in the trash didn't transform the contained emotion. Ripping the pages to shreds helped dissipate it, but the letter content demanded transformation. I concocted a ceremony—a ritual burning. Gripping the metal waste can in one hand, a book of matches and the stationery in the other, I scuttled out the back door of our fourplex rental to the cement patio, centering the empty bin on the slab, tossing the matchbook beside. With one index finger raised, I checked the wind speed and direction to be sure my mini-blaze wouldn't spread. Satisfied, I held up the pages in both hands. *Rip!* One tear down the center. *Rip! Rip!* Shreds of papers. *Rip! Rip! Rip!* Streamers stripping into ribbons, ribbons tattered into confetti, all scattered into the receptacle. Hands free, I snatched the matchbook, tearing out one red-tipped stick, sparking it along the flint edge. *Fwoosh!* A tiny flare emblazoned the tip, a hint of sulfur dioxide swirled in my nostrils, and I cupped the flame, dropping it atop the open kindling. *Woosh!* Little flames scattered, sparks singeing edges and igniting scraps, releasing smoke signals of transformation, burning anger to ash before my eyes. The charred remnants, flimsy crumbs of blackish soot, held no energy. Every flare of anger spent, the phantom effigy of my pain vanished into the air.

Weeks later, I tried another safe anger outlet Ms. Lynn recommended. One afternoon, on a stony shoreline, I gathered large rocks, piling them beside the river's edge. Grabbing a rock, I assigned it an injustice, a violation, or an outrage, thus naming my fury, voicing it, and hurling it into the air, thrusting it across the rapids, plopping it into the glistening waves with a gratifying *kersploosh!*

To the Dad rocks, "Stop lying to me!" *Kerplunk!* "Stop lying to yourself!" *Kersplish!* "Stop lying to everyone!" *Kersplash!*

To the Mom rocks, "Yes, I still think the incest happened!" *Sploosh!* "Yes, I know you knew about it!" *Splunk!* "I don't know why you don't remember!" *Splosh!*

To the rapists' rocks, "Fuck you, assholes!" *Kersploosh!* "How dare you rape me!" *Kerplunk!* "Damn you all to Hell!" *Kersplash!*

Each throw depleted the arsenal of abuses waged against me, until there were none left to name. My rock stash gone, I panted by the water's rim, exhausted and exhilarated, and I embodied the release of spent anger for the first time. My body, heavy-laden when I trekked down to the river, felt light and free as I waltzed back up the grassy bank.

After that big release, I started jogging as an exercise regimen again. My headphones blasted the *Chariots of Fire* title track and, with every strike of my shoes on the pavement, I imagined successfully fighting back against my rapists, defeating them, and running my victory lap. This physical outlet using imagery gave me the idea to angry-dance in my living room (channeling impromptu dance moves to emote rage), this time blasting Tori Amos, "Crucify," "Cornflake Girl," "Precious Things," "Little Earthquakes," and more. All of Tori's songs spoke to my soul, and she became my healing anthem artist.

The scariest anger outlet for me to attempt (one that my psychotherapist recommended) was to enact a tantrum—on purpose. I thought of my dad's vocal tirades as tantrums, as well as my teenage rebellions. In my childhood experience, Dad's tantrums ended with my dad leaving, threating not to return. And in my teenage experience, my tantrum fueled Dad's tantrum, and we two combusted. I slammed a door; Dad slammed me. My privacy. My protection. My door. All stripped from me.

The out-of-control rage proved physically and emotionally damaging to me. For these reasons, I was afraid to engage the practice. The tantrum technique Ms. Lynn described for me to try was not just yelling, but flailing on my bed, kicking and pounding the mattress, and beating the pillows. It was not a difficult thing to do in and of itself but was daunting for me with my history of tantrums, and besides, mature adults didn't act out this way, did they? Apparently, some did, in the privacy of their own homes. I joined their ranks. Adult tantrum-ers, unite!

My best tantrum involved two tennis rackets. I never had the notion to physically resist my dad. Avoid, yes, but physically deny him or defend myself, no. He groomed me to be complacent, cooperative, quiet—to just go along with his illicit advances without complaint, as if father-daughter incest was as normal as the two of us playing a hand of Go Fish. Now, as an adult, still harboring the seven-year-old and younger victims (the nesting doll selves, the combined early aged incest victims), I could fight back, with them and for them, against him.

I summoned these parts of myself that were hurt by Dad, the feeling of my skin crawling with his touch, the stuck feeling of being trapped with him between the sheets, the feeling of terror the night Mom caught him on top of me.

With these memories fresh, I breathed like an amped-up prize fighter ready to step into the ring. Armed, tennis rackets at the ready, I firmly clutched the end grips in each hand, then tested what it felt like to hit the first two strikes on the double bed mattress, giving the bed a one-two, *thud-thud*. Again, right-left, *thud-thud*. Four thuds, then eight thuds, and then my voice rose in sync with the drumbeat, "Bad Dad! Bad Dad!" Each right-hand strike was *Bad*. Each alternating left-hand strike was *Dad*, and the strikes quickened without pause into a frenzy of *BAD DAD BAD DAD BAD DAD*, and then the emphasis seamlessly landed heavily on the left hand, altering the chant to *DAD BAD DAD BAD DAD BAD*. I reclaimed my bed. I reclaimed my bedroom. I reclaimed my body.

I reclaimed my autonomy. Each wallop, each word, gave me back my power. My rhythmic mantra crescendoed with an accelerando, finally hitting a fortissimo sforzando. Resounding silence. The reverberation of my ousted anger shimmered in the air then mingled with my audible panting. Anger was no longer my enemy nor my greatest fear. I didn't have to hide it, or bottle it up, or eat it. I had a newfound respect for the power of anger and complete mastery of its safe release.

The culminating result of expressing my anger in healthy ways was composing more music. Angry songs birthed in the same way the sad ones had been.

"Joyride" on guitar came first and recounted my rape at age 13. The minor chord rhythms of the intro created a scene of suspense-filled motion. Mirroring the same rhythm, a melody filled my head and repeated until I could align words about the actual events into a lyrical ballad. From there, a chorus formed to bridge the verses together. After "Joyride" on guitar, two additional piano songs emerged.

"Thinner," another slice-of-life narrative (although more veiled), recounts the door-hurling incident of my final door slam. Again, a driving minor finger pattern in the intro provided a base of suspense-filled tension. This time, the lyrics came first, and I doodled a melody and chorus to fit them.

By the time I finished it, "Enraged," my angriest piano song, had channeled my power with a rush of force. But to start, I slumped over the keyboard, heavy hearted. Dredging up my buried rage was like digging up a grave, excavating layers of grief, examining the decayed remains. I scribbled words in my spiral bound notebook before touching an ivory key. A pattern emerged of four couplet phrases with a triplet at the end.

He'll flee from the danger he claims doesn't exist
He'll flee from the anger he claims doesn't exist
He'll get off with a slap on the wrist.
He'll get off with a yank of his wrist.
What are you running from?
What are you hiding from?
Don't you deny me my rage!

My doodling fingers fleshed out some D-minor chord progressions in a rhythmic 6/8 time, with the running baseline of a tippy carnival ride. The voiced melody arose on its own, a solo above the chords. The first four lines became the first verse, while the triplet naturally divided itself from the rest and, by adding repetitions, became the bridge and chorus. "What are you running from," repeated, as did, "What are you hiding from," together forming the bridge, leaving a triply repeated chorus to cast a spell of "Don't you deny me my rage!"

Several rousing rounds of unabashed singing of this beginning creation was enough to wear me out, like labor contractions, but the frenzied frenetic energy of the anger I was releasing propelled me forward to scribble two more verses—to complete an anger eruption birthed in song.

Just as my childhood piano tunes had soothed the Shadow Monster, my current songs soothed the exposed wounds no longer protected. My music opened me to express a fuller range of emotions than I had ever known. The compositions nurtured me to be well versed in my budding joy, in my deepening grief, in my desired survival, in my released rage. No longer shrinking from anger, my anger lost its power over me. I ruled my anger. I reclaimed my power.

After a few years of no contact with my dad, and much intensive healing work, I was able to forgive him. Yes, he violated me in unseemly inappropriate ways, and what he did was in no way condoned, but I still loved him. I reached out by writing him a letter of forgiveness. In my mind, it was my anger toward him that prevented him from acknowledging his wrongdoing. I naively thought that by extending my forgiveness with a promise of reconnection, he would feel safe enough to take responsibility for the abuse he perpetrated. It was my rejection of him that prevented him from being honest, or so I thought. His return letter was not the admission I expected.

Instead of thanking me, he wrote that my forgiveness letter was nice and all, but he had done nothing he needed to be forgiven for. I was stunned. It felt as if he had abused me all over again with this further denial. I felt more grief, knowing my father would never honor me by being honest.

It took me even longer to forgive him for rejecting my forgiveness. I had already grieved the loss of the father I'd always remembered at the same time as I had grieved the new-old memory of his incest betrayal. I had a further grief of a fresh loss of—again—cutting ties with him so that I could continue to heal.

The years of silence between us, minus this brief interaction, spanned a decade. At least I knew how to release my anger about this instead of enduring the molten lava in my gut. I waited until I was home alone, blasted the stereo, and gripped my two tennis rackets.

*I will sow seeds of self-nurturing
even amidst my despair,
so that when I weed out my despair
I will not dwell in barren ground,
but inhabit an embracing garden.*

CHAPTER 15

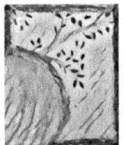

GROUNDING AND UNGROUNDING

My middle-management job waited for me, but I no longer wanted it. I loved and missed the people I'd worked with for the past eleven years, but the multitasking required to provide care services took everything out of me, without enough joy in return. Three months leave was barely enough time to scratch the surface of all the healing I had left to do. Even though I was doing better than I had been prior to returning to counseling, I needed a job that was less taxing—and perhaps not yet full-time.

I applied to the local school district as a substitute teacher and was hired. It suited me well at the time. If I was having an off day and needed to stay home, I could say no when they called me. Otherwise, I just had to get through one day at a time of someone else's lesson plans.

A year of subbing taught me that I did not want a classroom of my own as a career. I loved the kids and the teaching—it wasn't that—but the structural schedule and physical environment did me in. Some days there was no time for me to pee, and I held my bladder from 8:00 a.m. to 3:00 p.m. Lunch break: by the time I got my class through the cafeteria serving line, I had ten minutes left to wolf down my noon meal, which knotted my stomach. It just so happened that the classroom to which I was most often assigned was an interior room, with no windows to filter the harsh fluorescent lighting or view the outside world. I couldn't imagine the additional tasks—none of which I had to perform as a substitute—of grading, lesson plans, teacher meetings, and parent conferences, all fitted within the confines of the school day, which switched subjects every 40 minutes. My image from college—that this was my dream job—faded, exposing a potentially nightmarish occupation.

The school year ended, and summer vacation began. One Sunday morning, while faithfully filling my seat cushion at church, the perfect job fell from heaven—a part-time position working as a religious educator for my Unitarian Universalist congregation. The minister announced the opening from the pulpit before the Sunday service, and by the end of the coffee hour that followed the service, I had applied. Two more weeks and I was hired. I freely scheduled my own office hours, coordinated the Sunday School programs, attended a few evening meetings with the Religious Education Committee and the church Board, and then made myself available on Sunday mornings for the volunteer teachers, students and parents. I was already there on Sundays anyway, and now I would be paid. I was blessed to be surrounded by people I knew and loved, and it was a relief to have work that I found both spiritually meaningful and personally manageable. I devoted myself to the position with prayerful gratitude.

In addition to continuing my talk therapy, my own music kept singing through me, crooning tunes, including uplifting, hopeful songs. A musician friend had his first CD released, and, like him, I was anxious to record my music. Using the same studio, I professionally tracked all of the piano solos I composed in childhood, in the order that I wrote them. My first CD, just for me, I titled *Child's Play* and burned copies for a few family and friends. It felt good, inside and out, to celebrate the budding talents of the younger parts of me, parts that, despite tragedy, created tunes that soothed my soul. The album celebrated survival. Mine. Playing these songs over and over again helped me cope when I needed it—as I was growing up and into my adulthood. These simple tunes were like old friends. I had played them all of my life. Hearing them on a CD was surreal—my music existed outside of me, playing for all to hear, and I could simply listen and enjoy it.

The same studio recorded my guitar CD, *Every Little Piece of Me*. I finished the demo before I started performing so that if people liked my music, they could purchase a copy. I staged a few local, small venue gigs and sold a handful of CDs. It was easy to share my guitar music because—even though it was personal and spiritual—it didn't expose any family secrets. "Joyride" from this album detailed my rape, but it was less telling compared to the intensity of my piano music about the incest. I was not ready to record those healing songs for myself, let alone share them with the world.

My new job at the church began with a weeklong, on-site leadership training. Lay leaders from churches across thirteen states made up the 30-member class of adult students. It proved an incredible experience—in bonding with like-hearted people, in practicing interpersonal and group leadership skills, and even in gleaning insights into my personal strengths. I was delighted when I was asked by the staffers to join the training team.

The training team position required a three-year volunteer commitment as a trainer and planner. I hadn't even realized that all the staffers facilitating us for the week were volunteers. They taught like paid professionals. I accepted the position. Even though it wasn't a paid position, the church's professional training budget was able to compensate me for my time. I couldn't wait to offer the week's worth of learning experiences for the next three summers.

I had never experienced a more caring, committed, and talented group of volunteers as the people on this rotating training team. Each planning session and training week deepened our connections to each other. We'd say goodbye to former trainers and hello to new trainees each year, as our three-year terms were staggered to provide continuity to the training program. We covenanted to bring our whole selves to our meetings, and we created safe guidelines for interacting, paying particular attention to group process. It was a healthy framework we modeled for the students and practiced ourselves.

We staffers came to know each other well. It was safe to reveal our deepest experiences beyond our individual leadership talents. Everyone knew about my newly revealed childhood trauma and that I was navigating how to make peace with this unwanted narrative. I even shared some of my newest piano music with them that no one other than Kendal had heard.

My final summer on the team fast approached. And I devolved. It seemed recovering my trauma and reprocessing it in healthy ways was not enough to alter my brain chemistry. Depression blindsided me, and I gradually started back on medication after being med-free for three years. It felt as if all my intense healing work was for naught. Unsure I would be stable enough to attend the training week, I prepared to stay home, even if it meant missing out on a week that I loved, with people I loved.

I warned my teammates that I was not my best self. Possibly, I could have a manic episode during training week. Even though we were a well-oiled team, I could not promise to bring the high energy, focus, or attention to detail that was required of a staffer. I didn't want to detract from the learning experience or make more work for the rest of the team.

But everyone encouraged my participation. These beloved people thought the week would be better with a compromised version of me than it would be without me. I agreed to join them but gave them specific guidelines—be on the lookout for mania.

My college diagnosis of manic depression, or bipolar type II, was clinched with my hospital voluntary committal at age 21, when I swallowed the wrong pills, grabbing the tetracycline bottle instead of the Prozac in my suicide attempt. This first hospitalization, allowing me to peer behind the curtain of inpatient care, opened my eyes.

While locked on the psychiatric ward, a doctor was assigned to my case. This doctor had an impeccable reputation and was deemed the best psychiatrist on staff. I scheduled a meeting to talk with them about my discharge criteria.

Instead of meeting me privately in a consultation room, the white-coated doctor slouched opposite me on a corridor couch, which was lighted by glaring fluorescents and exposed to inmates shuffling past. Our space was pierced by laughing conversations from the nurses' station and invaded by a custodian mopping the floor. Annoyed but undeterred, I inquired as to how I could minimize my stay, requesting best-case scenarios and action steps to meet the requirements for my swift release. All the while, they (the doctor) looked at their watch, then gazed at the ceiling tiles, sighing heavily often, embodying utter disinterest. They interrupted me mid-sentence with, "I'm tired."

I stated, "I'm tired, too, but you get paid to help me."

For the first time, the doctor looked me directly in the eye and responded, "I get paid whether I help you or not." Abruptly, they rose and strode away—leaving me abandoned, my questions unanswered. Fortunately, the best psychiatrist on staff went on vacation the next day and was absent for the rest of my stay.

I asked the psych ward doctor subsequently assigned to me to take me off my medication, so I could start over with a clean slate. I reported that the antidepressant formerly prescribed, Prozac, made me brave enough, or numb enough, to try to kill myself. They scoffed, but I advocated that I was already safely in hospital care, so couldn't we try another approach? It had been so long since I was med-free, I couldn't remember what I was like when I was not chemically altered.

The doctor disagreed. They said I could refuse my meds, but they could not be held responsible for what happened to me if I did. I thought they were referring to my safety, which seemed odd to me, being under specialized care, on a locked ward, with padded room options and straightjackets available. Undeterred by professional disapproval, I stopped taking my meds but asked for an antacid instead. My stomach had been upset since I was admitted, and I was suffering digestive issues. Little did I know, instead of an over-the-counter antacid remedy as I was expecting, they prescribed an antidepressant that had a positive side effect of easing stomach upset.

I thought I was refusing my antidepressant medication. Instead, I was willingly and unwittingly taking another antidepressant in the guise of an antacid. The patients who had been there longer than I had warned that refusing medication could get me committed to a permanent mental institution. They had seen it happen to others who were no longer here on the ward, who had refused their medications and got a "free one-way paddy wagon ticket to the state funny farm." Could I be next?

To calculate my risk, I convinced a night nurse to peek at my file for me, to see if there was any notation of my medication refusal. The nurse confirmed that no, there was no record of me refusing meds. My relief flipped to concern when the nurse admitted that the doctor's antacid was charted as a prescription antidepressant. Though I was glad I was not at risk of being relocated as an uncooperative patient, I was concerned that my own best interests were being betrayed. I realized that the system didn't care about my preferred treatment options or whether I was discharged into my own custody or committed to an institution. I was just a patient. My case was all in a day's paperwork. Another release form to sign. It mattered not to them whether the paperwork dictated freedom or bars for me.

From that instant on, I role-played the model patient—polite, congenial, cooperative, compliant—and got out of the perilous environment as soon as possible. I reasoned I could do whatever I wanted, medication-wise, after being discharged. It felt riskier to experiment on my own, but I was suspicious of the motives and intentions of the doctors controlling me in the confines of the hospital. I did not trust them. It wasn't paranoia. It was realism. They had too much unchecked power, where I had none. The minimum stay for a self-signed-in suicide patient was ten days. I circled out the revolving door on day ten.

Kendal had committed me to a second brief hospital stay for a manic episode in my early 30s. The mania was medication-induced: I had an adverse drug interaction between my daily antidepressant dose and a short-term antibiotic. Fortunately, with that episode, I was under 48-hour surveillance and released without incident when the antidote they injected into my thigh brought me down to earth. I have had no more manic symptoms since.

Stress was also a trigger for mania. Even though the volunteer work with my colleagues for training week was good stress, it was still an intense engagement of my energy, which was significantly compromised at the moment. I gave my teammates specific behaviors to look for that would indicate I was manic. In a manic state, I would be unable to sleep, lose my appetite, lose track of time, and not be able to follow directions or complete assignments. I'd have extremely high energy and an overly positive outlook. If someone called attention to my mania, I would insist I was fine. The plan was simple. If I became manic, someone would take me to the hospital, even though I would resist going. I trusted them to follow through and felt hesitant—but safe—to attend the weeklong training session with them. Little did I know that I had just set myself up for potential disaster.

Friday and Saturday, the training team and I prepared for the training week. We arranged the classrooms and the worship space, got dorm rooms ready, assembled training notebooks, and ensured check-in would go smoothly. The students arrived Sunday afternoon. All was well, business as usual. Then Tuesday evening happened.

Each evening, a different student worship team was assigned to create a vespers service. The assigned team had free license to be as creative with that service as they wanted to be. The group assigned to Tuesday evening went all out. Their service theme was "Honoring the Child Within." They even chose to have the service outside in a flower garden amphitheater. They chorused "Teddy Bears' Picnic" as the processional hymn, with the worship leaders costuming themselves as oversized children, sporting beanies, suspenders, and pigtails. They skipped down the center path singing with abandon, some playing kazoos and tambourines, others blowing bubbles. The anything-goes mood was fun, lively, and carefree—giving reverence to play. The throng relaxed into informal worship mode.

The vespers presenters each shared personal and happy childhood memories. They invited the rest of us to spontaneously do the same. Several people rose in the crowd and regaled everyone with more childhood stories. Next, one of the presenters led a guided meditation.

In the meditation, we were invited to get in touch with a childhood version of ourselves. (Keep in mind, the seven-year-old and thirteen-year-old within me had already revealed themselves to me, and I had processed their trauma thoroughly in therapy and through my music. I considered myself at the other end of the healing spectrum as far as they were concerned. Nothing about my past was hidden anymore.) We were guided by the speaker to recall a carefree time when we were utterly and completely happy as a child.

I scanned and scanned and rescanned my memory and childhood events, including all of the non-traumatic ones I'd never lost. Suddenly, a tidal wave of grief washed through my entire being. A surge of tears welled up that I knew wouldn't and couldn't be dammed. Panicked, I rushed away from the service and just kept running.

I gasped to suppress my sobs and wails until I was far out of earshot. Then I crumpled, letting the grass catch and cradle me. I cried more deeply than when I finally identified my dad as my abuser, more profoundly than at Great-Grandma's passing. The grief that overwhelmed me was the grave realization that I had spent my entire childhood pretending to be happy. I knew I was supposed to be happy. I knew I should be happy. But the kid in me just wasn't. My heart broke for all of my younger years. A dam blocked me from my true happiness, a dam I could never surpass. Of course, some times were happier than others, but the happiness I experienced was always contained, my affect flattened, my gladness diluted, my delight watered down into something less than bliss. The deluge of tears collapsed the dam, flushing out the pain, cleansing the wounds, washing away the past, and my soul flooded with joy once and for all.

A couple of my staffer colleagues consoled me. By the time I wiped my eyes, I felt decidedly different. There was a lightness within me I had never before experienced. No—wait—not never before! I remembered feeling this lightness prior to the abuse starting, or at least prior to me deeming the Special Game as unwanted. The four-year-old me, untainted, felt this lightness. This lightness was indeed true happiness. My genuine joy looked like mania to my peers. The euphoric experience surged positive energy through my body, permeating my entire being. I knew it wasn't mania. Mania was scrambled energy, frantic, discombobulated, and confused. Mania made me feel disconnected from reality and anxious. This was the opposite. My positivity had core alignment and integrity to it. My energy was clear and very much connected to reality. I was genuinely happy!

Vespers was near bedtime, and I was wide awake with my happiness. I needed to sleep to get through the next day, so I did the next best thing I knew. I meditated. Not for five minutes. Not for an hour. I meditated all night.

In my mind, I was just going to sit until I got tired and then go to bed. The sun rose before my eyes, and I was still seated. I did not feel tired. The full night meditation passed in the blink of an eye. This experience felt like a download of source energy (a cosmic life force or a divine connection) streaming through my core. My mind's vibrational frequency was definitely altered, shifting from my usual consciousness of the material world to a supraconscious awareness of an invisible energy matrix that holds physical reality together. In Shakespeare's words: "All the world's a stage, And all the men and women merely players." In my heightened state of being, I got to peek behind the curtain to view the backstage magic that makes the play of life happen.

I imagined this must be what it felt like to be the Buddha. My eyes saw only love. My heart felt only love. When I looked into the mirror, I could see my great-grandmother's eyes from the other side, looking back at me, beaming with unconditional love. The world was a thing of blessed beauty, and I was part of it all. I felt kindred with the birds and squirrels, kindred with the sky and earth, and I felt like the sun's energy shimmered through me and amplified me like a mini sun. Rather than mental illness, my altered state encountered a spiritual truth, the oneness of me with everything.

Wednesday morning, everyone gathered on the lawn, our first group activity since the childhood vespers, and a few students led us in an ice-breaker game. The entirety of all of us formed a large circle facing each other, spread out arms-widths apart. For each decade of our life, we were instructed to—one at a time—take one step into the circle and say the most significant life event that occurred to each of us in that decade. If the most significant event was too traumatic to share, we were to simply say, "I survived," when taking our step forward. Of course, we stopped once we aged out, being too young to proceed any further into the circle, which resulted in the elders being in the center.

For ages 0-10, everyone had something to contribute: "Moved to a new school." "Broke my arm." "Parents divorced." "Baby sister was born." And so on. With incest being my most significant event, I stepped into the circle and said, "I survived."

For ages 11-20, others said, "Got my driver's license." "Met my first love." "Graduated high school." "Lost a grandparent." "Moved away from home for college." Not wanting to voice my rape, I said, "I survived."

For ages 21-30, more milestones: "Got married." "Got divorced." "Had three children." "Lost my job and found a better one." I wouldn't say "attempted suicide." It wasn't that I could not name my tragedies or share them aloud, it was that it wasn't appropriate in the context of this getting-to-know-each-other game. "I survived." I was not the only one to use the phrase. A few other voices also chimed in.

For ages 31-40, more of the same and other life events were stated. This would be my last contribution to the game, as I was still in my thirties. Now the most significant event in my life was the PTSD onslaught of my memories returning and the work to heal the wreckage. "I survived. And now I'm whole," I added.

Standing there, in my circle of my faith peers, I felt conspicuous in my honesty. No one else had four identical declarations like mine. Did others notice that *I survived* was my only response? I noticed and was astonished to realize how, in each of my life's decades up to that point, I had endured some form of major trauma. It would never have occurred to me—without playing this game—how difficult my life truly had been. It made me appreciate how far I'd come, how I was still standing, and how much more of life there was to look forward to, trauma-free (knock on wood, cross fingers, and pray to Goddess).

Yes, I was whole and one with everything, functioning within a higher vibrational plane. My brain was so macro-focused, it could no longer shrink back into the micro-focus needed to function in a human-constructed environment, let alone be a leader for others. Time wasn't linear, it was just now, always. I started losing track of time. My brain recognized words to pronounce them, but not to translate them into their intended meaning. The knowing I was experiencing was beyond words. I couldn't make sense of the day's agenda or follow along with my training notes. I wondered if this was what it was like to be an infant, full of cosmic knowing (an innate sense of interconnected eternity) and not yet figuring out how to engage this new finite state of human existence.

My senses heightened. I could feel when someone near me was experiencing physical or emotional pain. I didn't feel their pain in my own body, like empaths do, I just knew it to be there. When I noticed people with pain, I open-endedly asked them if they needed anything. They responded, if only they could get rid of _____ [insert ailment here]. Their complaints confirmed the discomforts I sensed. I told them I thought I could give them some relief if they wanted me to help them. Each time, the person agreed to let me give it a try. Intuitively, I used my hand movements and breath to clear whatever energy was keeping the ailment in place. Person with a headache—headache gone. Person with bottled up anger—anger gone. Person with upset stomach—upset gone. The sad person—sadness gone. It was miraculous.

Some people shared their positive healing experiences with others, and so more students sought me out. Each time I helped and was effective. Of course,

I wasn't making the blind see or the lame walk. I just had this novel knack for making minor symptoms go away. There was no explanation for either how I knew what was wrong with them, or how I knew how to relieve it. All this was going on behind the formal, organized scenes and in between training sessions. I had no former exposure to any kind of energy healing, not even in books. I didn't have a name for these spontaneous manifestations.

Fortunately, two colleagues understood I was having an ecstatic experience, having each experienced one themselves. They knew I was not manic; however, the rest of the staffers disagreed. After all, I was exhibiting all the signs I'd warned them about. They knew I hadn't been sleeping. At mealtimes, I was not hungry. And they saw me eat mostly bowls of watermelon. I was late to sessions, or didn't show up, because I was healing a student. When I did show up, I couldn't focus and perform. And I was amazingly happy. About everything. All the time.

Of course, I insisted I was okay and not manic, as I had told them I would. And I didn't want to go to the hospital, as I had told them I wouldn't.

If I were manic, the hospital would have been able to help me, with the same kind of shot I'd previously been given to bring me down to earth. I was not manic. The hospital could not help me with my ecstatic state. I knew I would be misdiagnosed and potentially harmed by being treated for mania while in an altered state of consciousness. That knowledge of the harm I could experience at the hands of good-intentioned, well-trained medical professionals was like the knowledge

I had about healing the ailing students. I just knew, without knowing why I knew. I was terrified to end up in a hospital. I wondered how many people committed to mental institutions were there because medical professionals misunderstood a peak experience. It frightened me to think I could be next.

The staffers who understood what was going on with me were heaven-sent. The majority of the team still voted that I should leave the training week. I agreed that I was making more work for the staff and causing them stress from worrying about me. Yes, having me leave was the best way forward. My angel staffers were able to help me advocate for having my husband pick me up and take me home, rather than sending me off to the local hospital. All agreed. If Kendal arrived and he thought I should go to the hospital, he could take me.

It was now Thursday afternoon. I started packing up my dorm. Buddha-me was going home. I would miss the last two days of the training week. I wouldn't be able to say goodbye to the students or to be part of the closing ceremonies for third-year staffers who finished their final volunteer rotation. This saddened me. I did get to say a bittersweet goodbye to my team. And I especially thanked my angels.

Soon, after arriving home in my celestial state, I crashed. Hard. My ecstatic peak lasted three days, and then as suddenly as it came, it vanished. The contrast was devastating. What had just happened to me? Where did that light-and-love energy go? Where did all of the knowing and innate healing retreat to? I experienced a different kind of depression within me. It was from knowing true ecstasy and then losing it. I wanted it back but had no clue how to make that happen.

Training week rendered me dysfunctional. Working at the church seemed impossible, even though I felt fully back to my human state. I had no trouble sleeping; in fact, that's what I did the most—all day and all night. My abilities to read, tell time, and follow directions all returned, but my motivation waned. My appetite came back, but all I craved were comfort foods. I had no desire to leave the house. The need to complete the paperwork for another FMLA leave of absence from work loomed over me. I could no longer perform my duties. I couldn't even show up to Sunday services. With the papers signed, I again had three months to regroup, without an income. "Here we go again," my defeat and worry moaned, haunting my thoughts. Fortunately, my professional care team was already in place and still active.

My private practice doctor knew me and my history well. I made an appointment and was able to relay the odd Buddha experience to them. They referred me to an acupuncturist.

Having never experienced acupuncture before, I was relieved that the needles used were hair-thin. I had pictured being stuck with inoculation needles. Instead, my skin surface could barely feel them being inserted and then lost track of where they were located. The acupuncture treatment itself helped release the pent-up depression energy. My body responded by quivering as energy released, vibrating into mild tremors on its own. I found it relaxing and energizing at the same time, but nowhere near my ecstatic experience. After my treatment, the acupuncturist introduced me to Traditional Chinese Medicine (TCM), teaching me about meridians (invisible energy pathways throughout the body), and Qi (the vital energy of the body), and gave me some Qigong exercises to do to enhance the flow of energy through my meridians. I even got some Chinese herb supplements, and we scheduled follow-up appointments.

When, during that first visit, I relayed my Buddha experience to the acupuncturist, they referred me to an energy healer. Despite my recent experience of spontaneously healing others, this seemed a bit bizarre. I didn't know people did this for a living. But, in my desperate state, I was willing to try anything.

The energy healer, a wise, older woman, looked like a kind grandmother, with gentle eyes and a loving gaze. She introduced me to energy healing originating from ancient India, confirming that my ecstatic experience was valid and not an expression of mental illness. She taught me about chakras (the seven invisible energy spheres located from the base of the spine to the top of the head) and auras (layers of invisible energy fields that surround the body) and how trauma could affect the body's energy field. Wow, was my energy stuck! Even though I now consciously remembered my traumas, part of my body's energy field stored the invisible energy of abuse, holding it in place, and it needed to be released. I vomited into a garbage can at one point, and all the energy healer had done was place her hands on my lower abdomen to free up the stuck energy in my second chakra, the chakra related to sexual health.

I felt the effects of her treatment instantly—a spaciousness in the pit of my stomach where I used to feel a knot, a knot that had remained even after my former ulcer had healed. The knot vanished! I thought back to the amazing results others experienced by my hands when I'd conducted spontaneous healing sessions at the leadership training week.

That week's mystery had an explanation, the miracle treatments had a guidebook, the marvelous results had a history going back thousands of years, and I was learning about energy healing for the first time in my mid-thirties.

I relayed my Buddha experience to the energy healer. She said it sounded like I was experiencing source energy, but I wasn't grounded, meaning the energy coursing through me had a greater connection to the cosmos than it did to the earth and my body. That's why I couldn't sleep and wasn't hungry and my brain lost the ability to read and track time. Perhaps I held an aptitude as an energy worker, she said. She showed me some physical grounding techniques, suggested some reading materials about chakras, and we scheduled follow-up sessions.

What I experienced after my energy treatment while at home was called a healing crisis. At the conclusion of our session, the energy healer explained that, because I had undergone such a long-awaited and dramatic release of energy, I might feel under the weather for a few days, as if having a cold or the flu. However, instead of purging a virus, my body would be purging the energetic congestion of the holding patterns in my second chakra I had acquired from adapting to trauma. In burying the memories of sexual abuse and subsequent emotional damage, I also buried the distorted energy present at the time of the trauma. The energy healer was right. I ended up needing several days to recover. I felt fortunate not to be working.

In between visits with my old and new health team experts, I devoured self-help books by new age authors, one after the next. The books I needed showed up when I needed them and reappeared when they provided me with new meaning, as if the literary world and the healing realm synchronized and synergized to assist me. Jack Kornfield's *After Ecstasy, the Laundry,* caught my gaze on the bookstore shelf just after my post-Buddha experience depression plunge. How handy! Then, I pulled Thich Nhat Hahn's *Peace Is Every Step* from my shelf and gleaned a new understanding of mindfulness and meditation since having my peak experience. How fitting! I eagerly read all the new age authors until they copied themselves by stating the same mystical truths in different ways. I sought teachings from world religions outside of my Christian upbringing, drawn to the messages of unity, light and love within all beings and of oneness with nature. I gained a new understanding of—and felt the experience of—the divine within me and within everything. This found grace was my source for healing myself in new ways.

Even with adding more holistic resources, I did not fathom that I was seeking advice exclusively outwardly, from the first hyperventilation doctors to the psychologists and psychiatrists, all the way through to seeing the energy healer and even reading the mystic authors. My assumption was that others knew better what was best for me than I did. I saw myself as a lost soul to be guided, a patient to be cured, a mental invalid to be fixed, a lesser being to be mentored by a greater one. After all, these esteemed others had the training, expertise, degrees, and credentials. I did not. If I followed their advice, I would one day be a normal, average, functioning human being, a regular person.

Then an epiphany struck—this time in a crisis of despair, rather than in a surge of ecstasy. I saw four experts in the span of a week. Unfortunately, or perhaps fortunately, they gave me four different and conflicting courses of action to best resolve my newest depressed state.

The first expert, a religious adviser, recommended going back on the medication I used to take, even though I had relayed that my body had rejected it during my Buddha state at training week.

Here is what had happened. Following the all-night meditation I did during the training week, I had had another sleepless night. At bedtime that night, I was deciding whether or not to take my antidepressant. I had been feeling so good that I'd forgotten to take the previous dose (on the evening of the all-night meditation). The medication was prescribed for bedtime because of its drowsiness side effect. I thought that taking it—though it was unnecessary because my depression was absent—might help me reclaim the sleep I had missed the night before. I swallowed the pill and climbed into bed.

Within 20 minutes of taking it, I felt odd. I began having tremors as I lay in bed. I was not moving my body—my body was moving me. The shaking reverberated through me from head to toe. Was I having a seizure? No, I could still think clearly, and move my body voluntarily. It was just that I was also experiencing involuntary quaking movements.

I called my angel staff people, and they came to my aid. One of them was a nurse. They knew what was happening and had seen it before. My body was rejecting a substance it did not need. My raised vibration was incompatible with the vibrational frequency of the prescribed chemicals. The nurse predicted that I would be fine, once the medicine left my system (in about eight hours). They were right: it did leave, and I was fine. But the night of shaking did not provide me with any real sleep, despite surrendering into the sensation. I was relieved when the shaking finally stopped in the early morning. The three of us did not relay my experience to the other staffers, as the situation had resolved, and we did not want to unnecessarily alarm them further.

So, back in my home community with my religious advisor, I had an ally seated in front of me that I trusted with my spiritual well-being, who knew the backstory, but still told me to go back on this precise medicine that hadn't been good for me just weeks before. For once, I felt like I knew better. Even though this person was not an MD, I felt betrayed, and for the first time, I did not take the given advice.

The second expert I saw specialized in a body trauma release technique that a girlfriend of mine recommended and swore by due to her incredible results. This therapy involved the practitioner putting their hands on different areas of my body—areas where trauma from all of the sexual abuse might be physically stored in the muscle memory. I wondered how it would be different from my work with the energy healer. When they described the technique specifics to me, I told the expert that I had already done these releases to myself intuitively during my Buddha episode.

Here is what had happened. During training week, amid my Buddha episode, when on an afternoon break, I went to my room to rest. While resting, I had the same intuitive knowing for myself that I did when encountering distress in others. There were places along my inner thighs that held fright. I gently placed my hands there and felt the energy of fear release out of my muscles as they tensed up, and finally let go. I did the same to my lower back and shoulders, where I felt the gravel dig into my skin during the rape. Again, tensing of muscles and then letting go. There was also gripping in my throat from all the secrets, long unspoken. I let out a long and victorious cry that felt like freedom.

This second expert dismissed my recounted self-healing experience, even though what I described was identical to how they would proceed with our session. In their mind, there was no way I could have done the technique correctly without specific training, and they told me so. I disagreed. I left the office promptly without the redundant treatment.

Expert number three was my psychiatrist. They told me it was too risky, with my diagnosis of bipolar II, to try anything outside of modern, Western medicine. Acupuncture and especially energy healing were out of the question. But, I asked, what about the positive results I'd already encountered? They called those placebo effects. They had heard claims of patients getting worse after energy treatments, not better. I was reminded of my healing crisis experience after my initial energy healing session (during which I vomited and was weak for three days afterwards), and dismissed the psychiatrist's concern for me.

The years of talk therapy and prescription drugs had only taken me so far. I was functional but not happy. In my mind, there had to be more to life than this. My psychiatrist reasoned that functional was the best I could expect, given my history and diagnosis, and that I should be glad because I was one of the lucky ones whose symptoms could be managed. I did not feel safe sharing my Buddha experience with this professional. I began looking for a new psychiatrist. Minimum functioning for life wasn't a good enough prognosis for me, in my opinion.

My longtime psychotherapist, the beloved Ms. Lynn, supported me in my exploration of the alternative healing realm. She had skillfully ushered me through the bulk of my healing once I remembered all of my childhood trauma. I aptly applied the breadth of her behavior modification skills and cognitive therapy techniques to process the emotions of betrayal, grief, and anger that enabled me to embrace the injured parts of me. It was a saving grace to find ways to navigate my family relationships and to find some peace within myself. However, the years of in-depth progress hit an impasse. I had reached a new stage of healing—applying the same techniques that had helped me come this far was not pushing me any further. I aspired to heal beyond what I had already achieved. It agonized me to say goodbye to this key person who, alongside me, had searched for my missing pieces, helped me cradle them in my arms, showed me my wholeness within my scattered parts. I deemed her as the sister I never had, but she had emptied her treatment toolbox with me. I bid her a teary farewell and inwardly acknowledged that therapy-wise, I was on my own from here.

The unfortunate-fortunate week knocked me to my knees. I cried more grief tears over giving my power away to other people. If my mental health were a car, I gave each expert a set of keys and allowed them to drive, steering me where they thought I needed to go, while I remained in the back seat, a passenger in my own healing, following their lead. All along, I should have been driving, with the experts riding along as navigators, suggesting possible routes, and me ultimately deciding which way to go. I recognized that these professionals, while experts in their fields of study, were not experts on me.

These experts knew what worked best for most people, most of the time, but they didn't know specifically how to concoct my best remedy or enact my best solution. They helped people and had undoubtedly helped me, but they couldn't fix anything or fix me. They were just human, and not the superheroes I'd positioned them to be. No more handing over the keys. No more pedestals. No more capes. My new mission—to save myself.

Letting go of this "someone will figure out how to save me" fantasy was devastating. It was equally brutal to know that dutifully doing what was asked of me by the experts was no longer the answer, at least not my complete answer to the question of how to be happy. Not happy in general, or happy enough, but happily me. Happy, like the four-year-old I rediscovered a few months ago in those brief, blissful days as Buddha at training week.

Just like before, when my FMLA was over, I did not return to work. Was it irony or full circle kismet that my position at my church both began and ended with the week of lay leader training?

More financial instability. Kendal voiced concern that we could not afford for me to be unemployed. He was right. We now had house payments. Credit card debt funded my mental health treatments with my first FMLA, when the forgotten memories surfaced. We had since paid off the debt. It was time to risk credit card debt again, assuming we would be able to pay it back or file for bankruptcy.

I saw this financial risk as an investment in our future, adamant that we could not afford for me to be sick for the rest of my life as a barely functioning human teetering on the edge of sanity. I needed to focus on my wellbeing with no external obligations, no distractions, with me as my own test subject, with self-healing as my full-time job, with me acting as my own heroine, figuring out how to save myself.

I am sitting...
    Sitting
        on my hands,
    Sitting
        on my heart,
    Sitting
        on my dreams,
Waiting...
    Waiting
        for you to stop talking,
    Waiting
        for the scenery to change,
    Waiting
        for the end of my days.
I am on the edge of my seat
    struggling to remain motionless and seated
        while being pushed from beneath.
    My posterior cushions me
        from possibility and pain.
    You may admire my chair
        or the way I am perched.
But,
    it is a perilous ruse,
Wanting...
    Wanting
        to rise,
    Wanting
        to topple my chair,
    Wanting
        to walk in my shoes.

CHAPTER 16

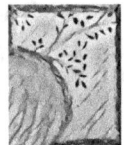

THE WOUNDED HEALER

I hired my four-year-old self as CEO in charge of navigating my healing journey. She held the compass, pointing to what made me genuinely happy, knowing how to reactivate the joy of living. The flood of tears at training week released her, spilled her onto my path, and when the water receded, returned her to walk with me. I longed to access her spark of light, like a flashlight leading me out of the darkness. This authentic version of me was innately full of glee within herself and of wonderment for the world. She embodied my pure essence, my before-the-trauma essence, the essence gone missing when I left the horrific memories behind—and inadvertently left her behind as well. While I kept trying to outrun the trauma, I had no way to know that that child filled with potential was pursuing me, wanting to take up her rightful place in my heart. In my toppled state, she overtook me, and I was ready to rediscover that good essence, to embrace her innocence, to reclaim that self.

The odd thing was, as Kendal noted when I took over my own healing journey, it looked like I was "just" playing. Indeed, I was playing. But for me, as an adult, playing was work. Even though I was doing things that looked like fun, I had to drag myself to play along. Part of healing was just getting me out of the house and interacting with other people, without the pressure of performing for a paycheck.

I had been replicating yoga positions at home with a DVD routine for several years. Afraid to attend a class in person as a novice, self-conscious about not knowing what I was supposed to be doing, I leaned on the DVD tutelage to bolster my confidence with the terminology and poses, making them familiar. Eventually, I got brave enough to sign up for my first class. In public. With others.

The instructor was a master of the mind-body connection. This was not competitive exercise yoga that had been mutated by the Western fitness crazes. This was mindful attention to my breath and body sensations within the poses, adapting the positions to suit me, feeling my joints and muscles, listening to emotional signals, being compassionate and gentle with myself, all the while stretching and strengthening the essence of me. The sessions included poses for enhancing each chakra's energy flow. Yoga class was my job, on my mat, twice a week for an hour.

A group of women met weekly for a day of painting. Class met from 9:00 a.m. to 4:00 p.m. Bring your own lunch and supplies and whatever you are working on. I hadn't done art since junior high school. The four-year-old me wanted to draw, so, following her orders, I joined.

Some dabbled in watercolors, others smattered in oils or acrylics, but I puttered in pastels, the closest medium to adult crayons. I treasured the memories of coloring alongside my great-grandmother, and the luminous sticks summoned her alongside my paper.

The instructor tutored me with the basics. Using primary colors, I blended a palette of oranges, greens, and purples, adding the tints and shades between, forming a color wheel. My next assignment was sketching a still-life apple, yellow and round, with a plucky stem, a shiny highlight plumping to the top right, a shadow casting left and behind, followed by vase of sunflowers, a rolling hillside against a sunset sky, and the harsh lines and sharp angles of original abstract designs—I wouldn't call myself an accomplished artist, but my work wasn't half bad. I spent the day being enthralled in the process, keeping my four-year-old happy with job number two, making art.

I saw a new modern dance workshop advertised to adult women of all ages and any level of dance experience. Not since college had I been in a formal dance studio, when I took ballet and modern dance classes for PE credit. Before that, I hadn't formally danced since switching from ballet to gymnastics in elementary school. Here I was in my thirties. The four-year-old me from yesteryear loved to dance, so I showed up, ready to move.

Over a dozen women joined. The instructor, twelve years my senior, was a professional dancer and choreographer with her own company. We met for an hour and a half weekly through a spring semester, learning choreography and creating our own individual and group dances. We prepared to perform on stage for an audience at the end of the semester.

It was a stretch for me and the other amateurs, reenacting our former dancer movements, reclaiming physical flexibility and stamina, learning new and complex routines, not to mention remembering the choreography and stage directions, but we were all in this together. Some of our dances would be interspersed with the professional company dancers. When it came time for the dress rehearsals, I experienced a thrill of adrenaline, rather than stage fright—my love of dance and joy of performing had been reembodied in me.

We fifteen barefooted women costumed ourselves in flowing tops and skirted pant legs, each sporting our own hue of a vibrant solid color—mine purple. On the night of the performance, the rainbow array of us huddled shoulder-to-shoulder backstage and encircled our arms around each other for our group hug pep talk before breaking to spread ourselves across the darkened stage, veiled behind the curtain.

From under the stage skirt, the house lights faded to black and the crowd chatter stilled to a few coughs and throat clearings. My late-30s-modern-dancer self felt as exuberant as the four-year-old ballerina at her first recital, waiting for the curtain to part, for the spotlights to beam, and for the music to start. Both energies intermingled within—the youngest performer I had ever been with the oldest one now on stage—ready for a tandem duet in a single body.

As the lights and music dazzled the stage, our bodies swayed, reached, and collapsed during the unisons and canons. Entering and exiting from upstage right to downstage left, in streaming lines, we dancers rolled, leapt, joined into shapes and dispersed again. The duets, the trios, and the solos ended in a finale with the whole company on stage.

The 90-minute performance seemed to end as soon as it began, time being like my Buddha experience, always now. As I bowed with my peers to the applause, cheers, and whistles of the relit audience, I gazed at my mom seated next to Kendal, smiling at me. She had never missed a dance recital. It still held true and included eight additional spring performances—my mom, always there, every year. The more I mastered wellness within myself, the closer my mother and I became. Even though she still didn't remember, she honored my memories as if they were her own. We got a second chance at the mother-daughter relationship we both had always wanted, getting closer to realizing it with each visit. We especially giggle every Christmas when we don our matching apparel—our penguin onesie pajamas.

The dance workshop was a spring-semester-only offering. I had to wait through the summer, fall, and half of winter to do it all again. In the meantime, the dance instructor offered a free, drop-in dance workout class so we could stay in shape until we met again for the next annual workshop. I sporadically attended the workouts. A few weeks later, I decided to host an informal dance class of my own—free-form movement to music, spontaneous, unchoreographed, inspired by my impromptu dancing at the lay-leadership workshop, the first year I was a trainer.

During that first summer leadership training week, I had jogged at sunrise. My route took me across a bridge over a spillway and along a river walk. Midway through the paved trail, a large expansive plaza overlooked the rolling river water and provided both a splendid opening to view the dawn and a perfect arena to dance, I thought, if I dared. (Other than my angry-dancing a few years back in the privacy of my own living room, I hadn't danced in years.)

The next morning, as I set out on the river walk, I took my own dare. It occurred to me that I didn't really enjoy jogging, but what if I danced two miles, instead? I had the freedom of being in a public space where I was otherwise unknown, out of state, and anonymous, and the few here that did know me already loved me. I jogged to music anyway—would it be so hard to skip, gallop, sashay, and leap instead? It turned out it wasn't hard for me at all.

Ah—the fun of it! Tossing my cares in the breeze, I almost lost track of how conspicuous my spontaneous choreography must have been to the few traditional walkers and joggers approaching, sharing those wee hours on the trail with me. When I reached the plaza, it became my stage for an exuberant free-for-all dance to salute the rising sun. I looked forward to returning to my sunrise stage, if only for the rest of a week. The last morning, after completing this new ritual, a kind, elderly man stopped me. He paused long enough to say, "It does my old heart good to see you dance."

Back home, I found another stage in the parking lot of a neighborhood park. I'd jog there, dance, and jog home. But too soon, the weather changed from warm moist sunshine to cool damp cloud cover, and when the winds blew snowflakes from the north, my outdoor sanctuary was blanketed in white and closed for the season. The church had a hall, vacant, sitting empty throughout the week. What if I could dance there? With permission granted, this hall became my private studio whenever the mood struck me.

A friend from the formal dance workshop, who was also a member of my church, heard about my dancing free-for-all and asked if she could join me. Of course, she could! That's when it occurred to me that I could invite others to join us, as well. I did. They came. I was not teaching dance to anyone. Rather, I was offering a time for people to move however they wanted to in the sanctuary space. No choreography. No routines. Just self-expression in whatever form that took. I provided the music; they provided the movement. It was an hour once a week that I could look forward to and a responsibility I could successfully fulfill. Another job perfect for me—dancing.

A SoulCollage® art class flyer on the church bulletin board caught my eye, and I signed up for it. This specific collage technique allowed a person to intuitively select images to create cards that then become symbolic reflections of that person. One could create many cards to form a deck of all the different aspects of one's self. In the process, the images would tell the unspoken story of what lies beneath the surface of a person's public persona.

I took to cutting and pasting quite easily. There were thousands of images from books and magazines available to choose in the class, already ripped out and ready to claim. All the pictures were stunning, so arranging several onto a card to my liking made the final product even more intriguing. There was no way to do it wrong or to create anything but evocative art.

In the initial class, I made three cards. The first symbolized my teenager-self being healed, Emerging Teen-Woman. The second represented my concept of source, that some call God, that I named Ever-Being. And the third represented a person of great influence in my life, who helped shape me, my great-grandmother, Twin Soul. I couldn't wait for more classes and the chance to make more card clues for my all-about-me deck. Eventually, I created over a hundred.

Creating the cards was just part of the process. Journaling about the cards helped me go deeper. Sometimes one of my cards appeared, seemingly out of nowhere, with no tangible sense of belonging to any part of me. Over time, the meaning was gleaned through an in-depth examination, setting pen to paper, letting the card speak for itself by letting the images speak to me. Every card ended up belonging and represented another aspect of the person I called me.

Where my music compositions started the healing process, the collage cards completed it. I finally had a way to observe myself from the outside, in an objective way. The hurt and hidden parts were no longer lurking inside me but leaped out, teleported into an image on a card. The cards outwardly held space for all that I once contained. I could breathe. I can't stress enough how integral these cards were in completing my healing circle. In them, I was able to see the beauty in my brokenness and the resilience that I had always possessed. I could lift pain directly out of my person and put it on a card. I could also see, with new eyes, all the lightness and humor that I brought into the world. I looked at myself without cringing or shrinking. I embraced all of me, who I was, what happened to me, and who I was becoming. It was all in the cards—another job well done.

Meditation opportunities presented themselves. Growing up, it was hard for me to sit quietly by myself. I could rest on the piano bench, meditating by playing the piano in the house alone, or I could straddle Dawn bareback, stopping time by riding my horse solo through the fields. Those were both respites in solitude, but not quiet time. I was actively engaging with music and nature beyond just sitting still.

Throughout my growing-up years, I thought I was an extrovert because I craved time with other people. What I was really craving was a distraction from being quiet by myself. If I was alone and still, I might be haunted by the Shadow Monster, feel brooding sensations I could not explain or tolerate. If I did find myself alone, without access to music or nature, TV was my main distraction, chuckling along with the canned laughter while cuddling with my dog, Tramp, or cat, Smokey, for company.

When I started working the church job, I joined a meditation group that met for an hour once a week. The sessions began and ended with silent meditation. In between, we discussed an assigned reading and shared personal insights. The book we deliberately unpacked, word by word, phrase by phrase, section by section, was a simply written, mindfulness text by a Vietnamese Buddhist monk, Thich Nhat Hanh. I loved the simplicity of his writing and his easy-to-follow examples of how to meditate and how to practice mindfulness in daily living. Both meditation and mindfulness could be achieved, he said, by paying attention to the present moment, focusing on what is happening now, rather than allowing the mind to wander and think of past events or future concerns.

Then, due to this community practice and this book, I could be quiet. It helped that I had already remembered and processed my past trauma prior to attending the group. In meditation, I learned to observe my thoughts without judgment and then to pay them no heed. Soon, I was enjoying vast moments with no thought. This foundation preceded the Buddha all-night meditation experience and helped steady the next stage of my healing, after crashing.

Later, when I was fully in self-healing mode with my four-year-old in charge, my meditation changed. I'd previously used meditation to help me forgive my mother, and my father—twice (first for the act and then for denying it happened), and to forgive my perpetrators. The person I had yet to forgive was myself.

It might sound strange that I needed to forgive myself. For what? I didn't do anything wrong. Happenstance and other people did me wrong. What was there to forgive having to do with me?

Children tend to blame themselves when they are abused. I did. Victims often blame themselves when they are raped. I did. For me, in both instances, I was haunted by what I coulda, shoulda, if-only-I-woulda done. But this was just the surface layer for me.

There was a deeper resentment lurking in my child-self and my teen-self about how I chose to handle my abuse in order to survive. With each trauma, I was put in a no-win situation. I opted to sever these two wounded souls from me by locking them away from the world and forgetting about their existence. Regardless of the fact that I was only aged seven and thirteen when I was coping with the dreadful attacks on my body, regardless of the fact that there was no safe place in the real world for both my everyday life and my trauma to coexist, regardless of the fact that the actual traumas were caused by others and beyond my control—the end result was the same. I had left the imprisoned selves alone, abandoned, without tending to their open wounds. They held me accountable for being their jailer. Which I was. That I was their jailer was the only truth that mattered to them in relationship to me. The outward circumstances did not negate the end-result damage from my poor coping actions, in spite of the fact that I had no other choice.

My meditations became sobbing events, rather than stillness and bliss. I heard my former captive selves cursing me, felt them hating me, and I understood why. My wounded selves outnumbered me, two against one; the child incest survivor and the teen rape survivor joined forces to gang up on the late-30s adult me. With every verbal attack they hurled at me, my mantra became, "I know. I'm sorry. I love you. It will never happen again." Over and over and over, this was my defenseless response to the fury, to me raging against myself.

In my meditation sessions, I consciously held space for all the wounding caused by my coping, coping the only way I knew how. The damage was done—not just by the perpetrators, but by me. I had to embrace this fact and acknowledge the suffering of my own making that I had endured. The only way forward was to have faith that the injured selves would forgive me for hurting them in my attempt to quell the pain of our original communal wounds.

Not so fast, the twenty-one-year-old me chimed in. Now it was three against one. *If it weren't for all the forgetting, I wouldn't have had to cope by creating mental illness symptom distractions that led to my suicide attempt that almost killed us all.* "I know. I'm sorry. I love you. It will never happen again."

Three against one escalated to four against one, as I heard from the most recently traumatized early-thirty-something self. *If it weren't for all the forgetting, I wouldn't have had to endure the night terrors and panic attacks that came with remembering, not to mention the job losses.* "I know. I'm sorry. I love you. It will never happen again."

These four distinct parts of me eventually vented all their frustration, spent all their anger, exhausted all their blame, and eventually soothed every hurt, stilling their if-onlys and regrets. When they were done, it was their turn to sob. I just held them in loving meditation as they bawled inside me, comforting them the way I always wished I had been comforted, but never was. I made up for lost time. I mothered and fathered all these parts of me within my internal embrace.

I didn't look forward to my daily meditation during this intense healing period. Some days I could only handle ten minutes. Other days I endured an hour. Those were my minimum and maximum allotments. The wounded parts of me knew that I would meet with them each day, and the rest of the time, they had to wait to voice their concerns. These established boundaries were the only way I could keep my days manageable without constant internal disruption. If they complained out of turn, I acknowledged that I heard them and assured them we would wait to discuss whatever it was at meditation time. And we did.

The consistency of my meditation and the repetition of my mantra, *I know, I'm sorry, I love you, it will never happen again,* finally paid off. All of my disparate parts softened, relaxed, trusted me again, and even believed I loved them unconditionally. And I knew they loved me back in return. I reclaimed the personal unity I had with myself when I was four, adding distinct extra parts: the 7-year-old, 13-year-old,

21-year-old, and early-30-year-old. With these additions, there was more of me to love. Now, the child could play spontaneously, the teen could explore curiously, the young adult could daydream peacefully, and the woman could breathe joy. These parts of me were now forever freed from making mature decisions, set free—carefree. They had permission to just play and have fun with no responsibilities. To just be. I created an inner sanctuary for them to reside. Deep within my heart, I imagined a tropical beachfront: white soft sand, gently lapping ocean waves, a blue sky, a few palm trees with hammocks strewn between, seagulls calling, warm sunshine. The four-to-seven-year-old making sandcastles, the thirteen-year-old splashing in the waves, the twenty-one-year-old picking up seashells on the shore, and the thirty-something me relaxing in a hammock drinking pineapple-coconut juice through a straw out of a coconut husk, all sharing their own little paradise—and Great-Grandma watched over them. My work was done.

*I have faith in an embracing universe.
I trust that while I am here, and when I am gone,
The universe will continue its infinite cycle.
Whether the "I" of me ends up simply as compost
for Mother Earth to rejuvenate Herself from my former shell,
or the "I" becomes a release of spirit energy
expelled into the universal unknown,
I trust my energy will merge with all that is.*

CHAPTER 17

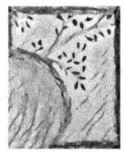

A TIME TO THRIVE

I knew my self-healing journey had found its true north when I got bored while playing. At first, it was hard work to play, then it became easier and more enjoyable. After excelling at playing, I finally got tired of doing only that. My wounds were healed, my inner selves happy. I wanted more. I was ready to move forward, to do something meaningful. My healing playtime spanned a year and a half.

The more I talked of being bored, moving forward, and wanting more, the more withdrawn Kendal became. I finally coaxed out of him what was the matter.

"You don't need me anymore. Are you bored with me? Are you going to leave me for someone better, for something better? What use am I to you now that you can take care of yourself?"

I folded this loving man—my devoted husband—into my arms and comforted him the way he had always comforted me. "I'm not going anywhere. I'm with you because I want you, not because I need you. You get to see what it's like to have a healthy wife for a change, a full partner. It's going to be different, but better. You'll see." We had endured the marital "for worse," and welcomed the "for better" now before us.

Both my Buddha experience and the positive results I received from getting energy treatments guided me to energy healing as my chosen vocation. I'd never heard of energy healing until my thirties, and it might have been useful for me to have been exposed to it sooner. I desired for more people to know about receiving energy work as a healing option. And I wanted to be able to offer the kind of healing to others that had been essential to recovering my well-being.

I found a school, The Eastwind School of Holistic Healing, two hours away. In addition to the holistic energy-healing coursework, I would also learn massage therapy—both therapeutic massage from modern Western medicine and shiatsu (acupressure massage) from alternative Eastern medicine. My formal training would incorporate the study of anatomy and physiology from distinctive yet complementary perspectives: from the chakra and aura healing of ancient India to the twentieth-century Japanese Reiki techniques of Mikao Usui; from the meridian lines and acupressure points of Traditional Chinese Medicine (TCM) to the trigger points and myofascial release of modern Western massage. Classes convened Monday through Wednesday each week, with a few weekend sessions that straddled Saturday and Sunday. It was doable by commuting, spending half of the week at school, and half of the week at home. The credit hours could span two years or could be condensed into six months. Being highly motivated, six months sounded good to me.

Logistics worked out well. So well, I felt divinely guided. I was concerned about winter driving. My term started in January and ran through June. The snow and ice storms blustered on non-commuting days. I was concerned about the expense of staying in a hotel while attending training. On the first day of school, a classmate offered to let me stay with them. Another friend of a friend needed an occasional cat-sitter over the weekends when they traveled for work. Their work travel and my workshop weekends happened to align. I had two new homes away from home with free lodging. I was able to attend all of the classes and complete my coursework on time.

Through the curriculum and assignments, I experienced more personal healing. In Reiki Level II, I was taught a special form of energy work, absentia healing (also called distance healing). The teaching strategy maintained that energy is universal and everywhere at once. A practitioner could summon the energy of a person far away to be healed, and that person still received a positive effect of treatment without being in the room.

After learning in class to perform distance healing as a group, we were individually assigned to use the same technique to perform distance healing for someone else. I fulfilled the expected version of this requirement and thought of another application.

I decided to do distance healing for my wounded seven-year-old self. I called her energy from the time and place of every incest encounter from first to last and rebalanced her energy field within those times and places. Visceral shifts stirred within me. I was no longer the jailed and the jailer, or the forgiver and the forgiven. I was instead the client and the healer. The outcome amazed me. Wounded energy I carried with me from the past to the present released out and away from me, leaving a vibration of healed space within. I experienced a lightness and a peace, like a sigh of relief. For the thirteen-year-old me, I performed another healing session, mending the rape trauma. I did the same for the twenty-one-year-old and the suicide attempt, and then the thirty-something panic attacks and the trauma of remembering it all. The energy of any part of my lifetime made itself available to me, upon request, and I could truly heal myself from the inside out.

Business classes were part of the curriculum. Even though I had no experience as an entrepreneur, I knew I wanted to work for myself. My tech-savvy husband helped me find a domain name, Wellspring Wellness, and launched the website using my design. A friend had a healing business, which included renting rooms to independent practitioners. I signed a rental agreement. A few business cards and brochures later, I opened for business as a massage therapist and energy healer.

From the beginning, I would have preferred to work from home rather than offsite. Our first house was too small for an in-home business. An eventual move provided the opportunity to find a new home with my business in mind. We bought a house with an office addition that had a separate entrance. I happily worked from home as originally envisioned.

Over time, I added more offerings to my list of holistic services. Three specific areas helped me reach more people and provide a wider range of healing options. Since the SoulCollage® class was instrumental in my self-healing, I registered for and completed their facilitator training. I was now qualified to lead classes like the one that got me started on those hundreds of cards (and still counting). Facilitating workshops was fun—both collaborating with my former teacher and seeing the new insights participants gained about themselves through making cards of their own.

Even though I took three levels of Reiki at the holistic healing school, I didn't take the Master Class (to learn to teach Reiki) offered a year later. It was too soon. I wasn't ready to be both a practitioner and a teacher. In a later class offered by my original teachers, I became a Reiki Master and learned to teach Reiki and attune new students to the healing energy. I enjoyed taking on this new venture of creating more healers, thereby launching more Reiki practitioners into the world. I was pleased to offer Reiki training to others at any level.

A friend had become a spiritual director and recommended her course, PrairieFire, to me. It was a three-year commitment, two years of personal spiritual development, and an optional third-year practicum to be recognized as a spiritual director upon its completion. I'd already taught a course (as a former religious educator) in creating one's personal theology. Since having my Buddha experience, I liked the idea of delving deeper into the mystical elements of all religions. I was also drawn to companioning others in their spiritual lives. I signed up and, upon completion of the practicum, added spiritual direction to my list of services. It became one of my favorite roles—to hold sacred space and provide deep listening for others.

My in-depth soul-gazing and the supportive people from my spiritual direction training helped me reach a place that allowed me to freely record and perform my healing piano songs. I collected them in an album I titled *Forgetting to Remember*.

After hours spent in the recording studio, the CD was finally completed and shipped for reproduction. My intimate healing songs were no longer too precious to share. Instead, they were too precious not to share. Soon, my box of CDs arrived.

Now I was ready to perform, on stage, in front of an audience. I sought local sponsors and donations to defray the costs of a performance. Many contributors stepped up with their time, talents, and dollars. This enabled all monies raised to benefit the women's shelter in town. My church provided the venue, the shelter staffers assisted with publicity, and I invited people from all walks of my life to attend.

Playing my songs repeatedly in my living room for the past fifteen years was my rehearsal for that night. I'd reached my late 40s, and it was time. Rather than stage fright, I felt centered and grounded. It was like a singing meditation for me, a soul offering from me to the audience.

The concert songs interspersed with my poetry, read by a friend, and complemented by my collage art on display. I began at the piano and moved to the guitar, ending on a high note with "Every Little Piece of Me," a song about communal unity. After a Q&A with the audience at the end, we all dispersed for cookies and CD signing.

The small venue (seventy persons, mostly friends) raised two thousand dollars for the women's shelter (between free-will donations and CD sales). The concert itself was a triumph for me, another layer of healing. I loved performing this concert and would do it again in a heartbeat. I relived the experience, many times over, in the privacy of my own home.

In retrospect, this night's success made me wonder what might have happened if my fourteen-year-old-self had said yes to the talent scout, had flown to California, had embraced the road to becoming a pop star. The agent had seen potential in my musical gifts that had only now come to fruition. Yes, I had what it took to be a performer, a singer-songwriter in my own right. Whatever success might have happened then, it could never have surpassed this one performance. I had something now that was missing then—wisdom within me—a truth to be sung.

Having already established meaningful work for myself that I loved through running my healing arts business, I continued to seek time to do some childlike playing. It was important for my four-year-old, who was still my CEO, to do things just for fun. The weekly dance group I hosted had continued to meet, and free-will offerings collected from the group's members supported local nonprofit organizations. I also hosted a drop-in lunch group that met weekly for friends to stay connected and well-fed and for a respite to recharge from work, family, and volunteer commitments. When I moved into the new house, a group of neighborhood ladies invited me to join them for morning walks. While our numbers had dwindled over the years, we'd maintained a routine of walking every weekday morning, weather permitting. These mini-communities reminded me of my childhood playground friends. I recalled recess being more important for deep connections with my peers than any class in school, and I have always thought that adults could use more recess time.

In my initial grief and successive expressed symptoms of mental illness, my great-grandma got lost in the shuffle. I didn't think to seek her where she was residing now, in a realm beyond the earthly one I still inhabited. I didn't think to communicate with her and feel her presence within me. The Buddha experience helped me to reconnect and remember her. I could often see Great-Grandma's energy reflected back to me in my own eyes when I looked at my face in the mirror. I felt her love and calm presence when I took the time to conjure her. I asked her to stay on the respite beach site with my many selves. She's been there ever since, and she brings each part of me the same comfort I knew when she was alive. Great-Grandma's being is present there with them. They can see her, talk to her, sit in her lap, and be soothed by her, and so can I. There is a little piece of heaven in my heart where she lives.

No life is without blemish, no person without pain and strife. As I write in 2020, I have more free time due to the COVID-19 pandemic. The seven-year-old and the thirteen-year-old are feeling aftershocks from our world catastrophe that are eerily similar to their experiences of being locked away from the world to survive. I reassure them daily that they are safe and loved, and this is a different, temporary circumstance. I must reassure my early-twenty-something self that survival is probable through self-isolation, and if hospitalization is required, it won't be like my first time in the psychiatric ward. My business is closed for now, except for doing a few spiritual direction sessions virtually. I remind my thirty-something self that this is not another job loss, that I will reopen and perhaps offer distance healing if the isolation is required for long term. I calm the present, unfolding version of me within the divine embrace of source energy.

As healing comes full circle, the parts of me that were once wounded tune their antennae and alert me if they see potential threats and dangers like those I've already endured. The difference is my various selves hold hands, we all trust each other, and none of us will be left behind ever again. We move forward together with unity, harmony, symmetry, a oneness that has endured since becoming bored with playing, since living my purpose, now for fifteen years, and counting.

I continue to live in the precarious form of a human being. But now, because I have found a place of safety and compassion for myself, I am open to notice my quirks and let them be, to recognize my missteps and apologize for them, to embrace my flaws and laugh at myself. Learning to take myself lightly (and not quite so seriously) continues to be a challenge for me, but I'm getting better at it. Do I annoy myself? Yes. Do I argue with my husband? Yes. Do I rail at the world? Yes. But that's part of my humanness, giving myself permission to start over, begin again, as soon as I stop being grumpy, and then repeating the cycle many times a day.

A popular saying is *all things happen for a reason*. If it refers to cause and effect, then I agree. If I hurt someone, intentional or not, they become injured. But when "all things happen for a reason" implies that bad things happen for a greater good, I disagree. No one deserves to be abused. Not everyone survives their abuse or the turmoil thereafter. Are those who don't make it any less deserving of healing? No.

If I had grabbed the Prozac as intended, my suicide could have been complete, my possibility of healing obliterated, and this book nonexistent. Everyone has a story that deserves to be told and heard. Everybody injured has a right to heal and live a fulfilling life. Those of us who survive and heal are not inherently more worthy than those who do not, and it's not about making better choices or having a keener skill set. There are no choices in the lose-lose situation of sexual abuse. There are no skill sets to prevent perpetrator violation, overthrow their trespass, or reverse the damage they inflict. Blaming and shaming victims before, during, or after abuse occurs imposes further injury. People are abused because perpetrators do harm, and, most often, the perps get away with it.

Can something good come out of it? Sometimes. I was lucky enough to experience full-circle healing, but I had other things working in my favor. Did I work hard? Yes. Was I determined? Yes. Did I take an unconventional route? Yes. But that is not the full picture.

I acknowledge my white privilege, living in a culture that centers whiteness. Racial injustice abounds out in the open for all to witness on social media. Another unarmed black man is murdered by a white police officer, with malice, in front of the world stage. When will "liberty and justice for all" include liberty and justice for black citizens? Answer? When we dismantle all that enables white dominance within our institutions. Then our society we will be closer to realizing equality.

In addition to being white, further unearned privilege includes being heterosexual, cisgender, able-bodied, and middle class. All of my physical survival needs were met with a few bonuses. I was able to attend college at a time when fees were not yet insurmountable. My extended family and key people in my life helped me through, like my great-grandma and especially Kendal, along with many others. Where would I be without them?

I had my music and my musical circles of friends, teachers, and activities. And there were my horses, along with the dogs and cats in my life, readily available for comfort. I had access to healthcare and a variety of mental health professionals, as well as access to credit debt used to fund my eventual recovery. For every story like mine, there are countless others who have overcome more trauma with fewer resources, and their lived successes have not been told.

I am also uplifted by my felt connection to a source of universal energy flow, my interdependence with Mother Earth, my interconnections with people, my communion with pets and nature—my own version of faith. It was important for me to adapt the teachings of my Christian upbringing to what I felt to be true in my soul. No single world religion I explored could describe what stirred within me, but they all had mystic teachers that touched my internal inklings. That's how I came to be a Unitarian Universalist, much to Godmother's chagrin. She would have deemed herself a success as a Godmother if I was regularly sitting in the pew of my original church, or, at the very least of my baptismal denomination, but in my mind, I hadn't gone astray. That foundation held me as I became more spirit-led, less indoctrinated, and better able to hear and listen to my calling.

Part of coming full circle for me was to be able to extend forgiveness beyond myself, beyond those three teenage boys, beyond my mom, to my dad. After forgiving my dad for the incest he subjected me to, I forgave his denial of it by agreeing to disagree. During my deepest healing, it hurt me too much to have a relationship with him. I needed time to heal by myself, on my own terms. That distancing decade was necessary to get out from under his shadow. It might have continued indefinitely, but something within me shifted. It hurt me more to not be in contact with him. He was part of my life beyond the incest.

A children's book explains how I had enough compassion for my dad to want to reconnect: *The Little Soul and the Sun* by Neale Donald Walsch. The story features souls in Heaven, and one little soul in particular who wants to be born on Earth for a specific purpose—to be the light of forgiveness. However, for the forgiveness soul's light to shine, another soul must be willing to be born on Earth, partnering with the forgiveness soul, providing an injury that necessitates forgiving. What other soul would want to lower its vibrational radiance enough to be the injuring party? It seems too much to ask, and the forgiveness soul assumes no other soul will agree to do the loathsome job of providing the injury.

A friendly soul steps forward and agrees to be the injuring soul. The forgiveness soul is so appreciative and grateful that thanks can't be expressed enough— for it is through the injuring soul's sacrifice that the forgiveness soul can fulfill its desire. The injuring soul needs the assurance that the forgiveness soul will indeed forgive, or it's not worth the sacrifice of becoming less vibrant. Their pact is sealed with a promise.

Through the process of being born on Earth, the forgiveness soul no longer recognizes the companion injuring soul but remembers the promise made: that the injuring soul would be forgiven. Indeed, while on

Earth, the forgiveness soul shines the light of forgiveness on everyone who causes injury, fulfilling its desire and honoring the promise made to the injuring soul companion.

This fairytale, figurative for me, provides a lovely metaphor of how to embrace those who have hurt me in the world. I would want to be forgiven for the worst thing I ever did. It's not about degrees of hurt, or intention, or even confession. I have found a soft place within me with no need for revenge. It does not condone the perpetrator or ignore the injured party. It acknowledges that our internal struggles can and do cause others harm. It embraces us all as being human.

I navigate my relationship with my dad very carefully so as to avoid further injury. He has neither acknowledged what he's done nor apologized for it. I show up as my full self, though he can only view a portion of our joint history, a small part of who I am. This prevents him from knowing or embracing the parts of me that have evolved from the healing I've done. I can understand his blind spots without dishonoring my truth. I cannot pretend that what he deems real is the whole picture. I have done too much healing work and refuse to sidestep my own power.

Even after forgiving my dad, it's hard for me to be with him. My wounds have healed, but he still harbors a wound of denial on his end. The incest denial is his wound, not mine. He cannot heal it because he cannot admit what he's done. I cannot heal it for him.

I believe the part of him he has conscious access to doesn't remember hurting me because he is the consummate forgetter. I don't think he would intentionally lie to me about that. But I think the part of him that does remember lives deep in a place he prevents himself from reaching—much like I knew, but didn't know, about my own parts that I buried. Whether or not he remembers is irrelevant. The open wound on his end is still there.

His wound is like a shattered windowpane, with shards of glass outlining the perimeter. He is unaware that he resides inside a house with a broken window, but I clearly see it. The jagged opening is the only way for me to enter his home, to join his world without renouncing my own. If I enter through the front door, the door he holds open for me, I would be pretending right along with him that the incest never happened. Instead, I must climb through the broken window, pass through the shards, each time I connect with him. It's risky and painful (as I invariably cut myself coming or going despite moving carefully), but it is the only way to join his world without renouncing my reality. I reach him by entering through his wound, and my dad and I reside in the shallows of what he remembers.

I have already grieved that he cannot go deeper. But I can honor the good that is also present within him, like the time when we were living in the new acreage house. Tornado warnings clamored over the airwaves. Distant sirens wailed. We, as a family, hunkered down in the basement with our dog Tramp. I cried that our pony, Cinnamon, would get blown away in her shed of a barn and pleaded with my dad to please let me bring Cinnamon in the basement with us. I would run as fast as I could, and it would only take a second. Against his better judgment, and despite my mom's protests, Dad rushed out, blasted by the fiercest of winds and whisked Cinnamon through the ground level sliding glass doors to safety, standing her over the basement drain. I thanked him profusely, overjoyed that she was safe, that we all were, and all was well. My dad saved Cinnamon from the tornado, which thankfully didn't touch down, and for a fleeting moment, Dad was my hero.

*Every little piece of me is in every little piece of you,
And in every little piece of everything.
And all I want to do is love every little piece of you
So that I can love every piece of me, in everything.*

Afterword

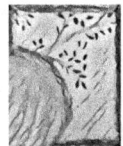

HEALING POTENTIAL ABOUNDS

So, what is healing? It is not the same as curing. Curing implies that the disease itself and the underlying factors that caused it are gone. While the Shadow Monster is gone, the underlying factors of my abuse remain intact. No cure will erase either the events or the coping strategies I activated to survive. My bipolar symptoms are in remission—meaning the ups and downs in my life swing within the range of normal now—but I take care to tend to these average swings in a preventive manner, knowing the hazards for me when they swing too far. I recognize when my body needs to recalibrate and take a personal sick day to rest and restore. If I were cured, I could ignore my subtle mood variations, but I know better than to let them fend for themselves.

If I were cured, I would have been able to finish watching *Dickensian*, a British television series aired on public television that featured some of Charles Dickens's most famous characters, including a young, eligible Miss Havisham. Having suffered through

Great Expectations, despite the forty-year gap and the alternate narrative, it was neither worth my time nor energy to expose myself to even the subtlest lingering reminder of the fictional creature.

And if I were cured, I would have no triggers. The triggers are fewer, further between, and less intense, and I tend to them when they arise, having learned to discern them in the moments they hit. This happened most recently when the US Center for Disease Control recommended people wear masks in public during the 2020 coronavirus pandemic. When I put on my mask for the first time, my facial muscles flashed a sensory memory of a sweaty palm covering my mouth. Rather than a wave of panic, a slight twinge was all I felt, and I stood fully in the present moment, reminding myself I was in the here and now, not back there and then, and eased my breathing into the mask to calm the thirteen-year-old within.

Tending to the slight variations in my moods, avoiding optional stressors, and treating triggers with awareness and TLC are parts of my ongoing healing. I've gone months without a single thought or reminder of my past trauma enlivening my senses. In the throes of healing, I didn't think I would ever be free from the relentless revisiting of wounds or the pain of them, but I'm grateful I was wrong. Time, space, and the healing thus far have put my past further behind me with each new day.

Numerous obstacles stood in my way along with the mental condition itself: financial instability with me being unable to work, insurance caps on the number of counseling visits I was allowed in a year, expenses not covered for hospital stays, mental health deductibles required to be met each year that were separate from the deductibles for general medical services, the bankruptcy risk of delving into credit card debt, the stigma of mental illness in society, and the biases of some care providers. It took time, persistence, tenacity, self-advocacy, and endurance.

All of this was required of me when I was functioning at my worst. It's a mystery how I managed it. Any one difficulty could have prevented my eventual healing. For this reason, when anyone begins walking upon the healing path, it is an extraordinary achievement—worthy of celebration.

The idea of fairness was a stumbling block in my healing process. I clung to the fact that what happened to me wasn't fair—the abuse wasn't my fault, and I didn't deserve it. It was maddening that the people responsible for hurting me took no responsibility in repairing the damage they had done. They hurt me. They should have to heal me, right? Why should I have to heal a wound someone else made?

But with time, I saw a bigger picture: why would I want the people who hurt me to be put in charge of anything having to do with me? They were clearly careless, unreliable, reckless, and damaging to my well-being and deserved no power or agency where I was concerned. They were oblivious to my pain, so how could they even begin to know how to treat it? I was the only person who knew exactly what I had needed and didn't receive at each point of injury. Because of this intimate knowledge, I had every advantage, knowing exactly what injuries needed healing within myself. My own tender loving care far surpassed anything the perpetrators could have offered, and my professional team of allies knew the way. The fact that I needed healing was unfair. That my professional allies and I are better suited to tend my wounds is more than fair.

It's been over fifteen years since I have consulted a mental health care professional. As times change and mental health diagnoses evolve, I've been asked by friends in the field who know my story if my Bipolar Type II diagnosis was the right one, and if Complex PTSD might be more accurate now. It's possible. At the time of my original diagnosis at age 21, I had yet to recover any memories of childhood sexual abuse. Later, when I experienced PTSD symptoms with trauma memories, Complex PTSD was a newer concept, and the term was not mentioned in my treatment plan. It gives me hope that the medical field discovers nuances in old diagnoses over time and finds new ways to help patients recover their well-being.

I compare healing to well-being and curing to health. Healing, like well-being, flows from acceptance and awareness of what is. I can experience illness yet have a feeling of well-being, just as I can experience health and feel ill at ease. The flow of acceptance in the present moment awareness can be at times frightening and at other times soothing—as frightening as acknowledging a panic attack while it's raging, as painful as recovering a memory of abuse, as difficult as grieving a living relationship that is beyond reconciliation. And it is as simple as noticing a beautiful sunset, as delightful as absorbing a sloppy kiss from a canine companion, as easy as inhaling the fragrance of a rose. Healing happens moment to moment, deepening my ability to hold space for the worst and the best parts of my life. The more I embrace both ends of the continuum, the more at ease I become overall. Tangible contributing factors intertwined with indefinable mystery to enable my healing. I am eternally grateful that my life has a happy middling. How did that come to pass? It was refreshing to find a psychiatrist who treated me like a human being with innate healing potential rather than as a permanently damaged patient. The professionals who most helped me understood I needed healthy coping mechanisms to replace my old survival habits that had outlived their benefits. The more widely my Western-medicine-trained experts embraced alternative medicine, holistic approaches, and healthy lifestyle changes, the more I benefited. In combination, these trained guides created a makeshift treatment team akin to integrative medicine to suit my unique needs.

For me, that treatment included reducing stress by practicing yoga and meditation, enhancing my body chemistry by changing my diet, adding vitamin and herbal supplements, increasing my natural endorphins by immersing myself in hobbies like playing music, dancing, collaging, journaling, gardening, socializing with friends, and lots more.

I no longer needed symptoms to distract me from my past stress—the secret trauma of my childhood—because there was nothing left hidden. I could deal with any new stress head-on with new tools and deconstruct it before it became a barrier to my health and well-being. And just as my trauma resulted from the misfortune of me being in the wrong place at the wrong time with the wrong people, my healing resulted from the fortune of me ultimately being in the right place at the right time with the right people.

My writing is inspired by three *Juicy Living Cards* by Susan Ariel Rainbow Kennedy (SARK):

"The book of your life is rare and marvelous."

"Write your life so that others may be illuminated."

"The tiniest story in your life can deeply touch another. You cannot know the effect your story might have."

These card sayings have been with me throughout my writing process, reminding me that it is okay and good to share my truth and helping me to be brave enough to keep writing.

I have shared my steppingstones with you, but I also offer a word of caution—one person's steppingstones can be another's tripping hazards. A dear friend, inspired by my healing journey, followed my footsteps, hiring my beloved counselor, taking a SoulCollage® class from my original teacher, and joining the women's dance workshop offered another year. She clashed with my counselor over scheduling issues, was thwarted by her collage images not fitting on the cards the way she imagined and was overwhelmed with the performance expectation of the dance workshop and dropped out. To her credit, she attempted new things outside of her comfort zone, and when they didn't work for her, she searched elsewhere and found her own steppingstones.

Healing looks different for each person and won't necessarily resemble my path. Reclaiming wholeness is an individual journey, and every person is unique. It is not necessarily about whether or not medication assists well-being, or whether therapy is or isn't part of living a best life. For me, the markers of success are enjoying the life I have and being comfortable in my own skin. Success is loving myself unconditionally, while keeping my ego in check. It's about recognizing red flags and avoiding the missteps that spiral me downward. It's about adapting to changes in my environment, be they internal moods or external stressors, and using the tools I have acquired to shift as needed for my well-being. A healing journey has stops, starts, retraced steps, occasional wrong turns and then right ones, and random wandering before detecting an internal compass. Others' healing paths, though perhaps parallel, will never look identical.

I reached a point where being me was so excruciating, I would have gladly traded lives with anyone. But now, I am thankful, there's no one I'd rather be than me. I have my past that sometimes whispers but no longer haunts me. I have my present that, even when challenging, is better than all that came before. And I have my future, and I lean into this unknown with more hope than hesitancy, more faith than fear, and more love than I ever imagined.

I hope you, Dear Reader, find something useful in the pages of my story. It is my intention to be a healing balm for others wounded by sexual abuse. I share my words as an offering of peace, hope, and love. May you hold these blessings as truths in your own heart.

Memorial Shells

*A squiggly line
a frame of mind.
Brainwaves like ocean tides
wash up skeletons on the shore
others call treasures.*

Acknowledgments

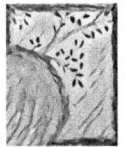

With Thanks, Praise, and Gratitude

Here are the people who got me through until I was able to find my footing on the stepping stones to healing. Each person is a point of light on my path, leading me back to myself and my happiness. Throughout my life, I have been touched by others and by their stories. I appreciate all who have crossed my path, those who previously walked alongside me briefly or for a time, and those who are still walking with me in body or spirit.

My constant companion in my adult years, through illness and recovery, has been my husband, Kendal. Without fail, he has been here when I most needed support. He is the mountain, and I am the wind that blows around the mountain.

My childhood besties (whether renamed—Erin, Lenee, Jodie, Mindy, and Justine—you know who you are, and other friends whether referred to or not mentioned) offered me, in my growing-up years, kinship that I still cherish. All my church, band, and chorus friends helped me belong and made teamwork fun and meaningful.

My two long-term boyfriends offered me love and welcomed me into their families. These loving families embraced me as their own. My college off-campus roommate, Ginger (Walter) Primrose, and her entire family kept me and still keep me on course, as a touchstone from my college years. Family friends Sara and Randy Compton leave their door and hearts always open, and I am eternally grateful.

To all my piano teachers, from my first to last: thank you for sharing your passion for music and championing my own. To my band teachers and my choir directors: you all made my life better with your talents and love of music. To my voice teachers, Julie Simson and Jean Thomas: thank you for taking a personal interest in me beyond my singing.

To the experts that were most helpful in their own fields: Ms. Klatt, LISW, ACSW; Dr. Carlson, MD; Ms. Stallbaumer, LAC, MSOM; Ms. Angelici; and Dr. Barloon, MD; I appreciate you listening to me, honoring my innate worth, and believing that self-healing is possible.

Everyone at Mainstream Living created an extended family for me for eleven years. I deeply appreciate your love, support, and generosity.

To Midwest Leadership School students and trainers, for both the adult and youth sessions: thank you for showing me through your presence what a loving community looks and feels like. To UUFA members and friends: you helped me transition to a healthy, spiritual place that I still enjoy. To the larger UUA community: you exemplify a religious body with a compassionate and wide embrace for all people and the planet that aligns my faith.

My energy teachers, Candida Maurer and Michael Santangelo instilled in me their wisdom and skill, which I use as a foundation for the healer I am today, and I am better for having been their student. To the Eastwind students in my class, thank you for being partners on a new path. I give special thanks to Anna Evans who welcomed me without reservation as a guest into her home, and to Sadja Pals my other home-away-from-home provider, both of whom made commuting possible and enriched the experience through knowing them.

To Ria Keinert and colleagues at HealthWise Resources and Keith Schrag and colleagues at our South Walnut healing center: thank you for providing space and support to help my business thrive.

To my PrairieFire companions, facilitators, and Sisters at Atchison partners: my life is continuously enriched by your opportunities to deepen my spiritual connection. To my Supervision Group colleagues: your presence is analogous to healing, and I look forward to our every meeting.

My life is graced with many kindred spirits. Lori Allen, I am fortunate that our paths intertwine, overlap, and circle back to reconnect. Deb Anders-Bond, you turned me into an artist. Kelly Poole, your playfulness is my muse. Betty Young, you always see the best in me. Donna Lutz, you teach me to glean the sacred in the tiniest of things. Amy Slagell, your groundedness and positivity keep me likewise. Ruthann Hadish, I aspire to your gentle peace. Valerie Williams, your dance inspires my own. Locky Schuster, you reminded me that coloring is ageless. Marsha Diggs, you'll always be my heart sister and monkey sister. Cheryle Tucker-Loewe and Mark Cummings, thanks for being there when it counts. Rev. Mary Jane Oakland, you are my divine intervention whenever we meet, and it is my honor to bask in your example of being.

My community groups enrich the present. Thank you, Compassion Circle participants, for strengthening my own compassion for self and others. Dance Be+Cause members, thanks for playing with me and providing donations to our community nonprofits. Lunch Ladies, thanks for showing up as yourselves and sharing. Neighborhood Walking Ladies, I'm grateful for connecting with the dawn and celebrating birthdays. Thank you to all the women in and out of the Women's Spirituality Group over the years that witnessed my journey with your listening. A special thanks to Women in Motion members who danced me to revival. And Transform Collective members, I appreciate your genuine interest in my story, so much so that you gave me the courage and motivation to write it down.

My musical friend Reggie Greenlaw, I treasure the introduction to Paula Brown and relish your harmonica improv on my Joyride song. Paula, it was a pleasure to record my childhood piano solos and guitar album with you. And to Dennis Haislip, your professionalism and expertise eased the process of recording my healing piano songs. You further promoted my fundraising concert, and I appreciate your personal encouragement of my music.

To ACCESS staff and volunteers who coordinated the HeARTs for the Arts program, The Clothesline

Project, and Sexual Assault Awareness Month events, especially Angie Schrek and Marcy Webb for their work on my benefit concert, you provide the community with excellent and much-needed services, of which I was privileged to be a part.

A special thanks to all who have walked through the doors of Wellspring Wellness, be it once or many times over. Your trusting me with your well-being is a gift each time I see you.

To my family members in all their forms, immediate and extended, by birth, marriage or choice, here and gone, thank you for being in my life. You dotted the calendar of my youth, and still do, with holidays and celebrations, giving me events on the horizon to look forward to. I am blessed beyond measure. And thank you to my parents. Mom, your support has grown alongside my healing, and I cherish our mother-daughter times together and our joint sense of humor. Dad, as we agree to disagree, we may not see eye-to-eye, but we still connect heart to heart.

Thank you to my readers, Suzanne Zilber, PhD, LP; Art Konar, PhD, LP; Jeffrey Means, MDiv, PhD; Diane Glass; Kathy Reardon, RN, MS, Spiritual Director; Candida Mauer, PhD, Deb Wiley, Nancy Jones, PhD; who added their suggestions to make my book a better read for service provider professionals and the general public alike. Your contributions benefit each person who reads my book.

To my editor, Ann Outka, thank you for finding the pesky errors, polishing my prose, and guiding me to be more specific, thereby making my story concise and clear.

This book would still exist only in my mind if not for professional excellence of Diane Glass and Mary Nilsen. Diane, thank you for your generous mentorship, guiding me through the initial writing process with your experience and expertise. My story is infinitely better from its beginning draft because of you. Mary, I appreciate your immediate interest in publishing me as a first-time author. You enhanced my writing by teaching me one-on-one from your book, *Words that Sing: Composing Lyrical Prose,* helping me to find my voice. I am grateful for your professional skill in navigating me through my manuscript draft to the final book product with ease and grace.

And thank you, Dear Reader, for your willingness to share some time with me by reading my story. May you bring healing full circle by sharing something that touched your heart within these pages with someone else.

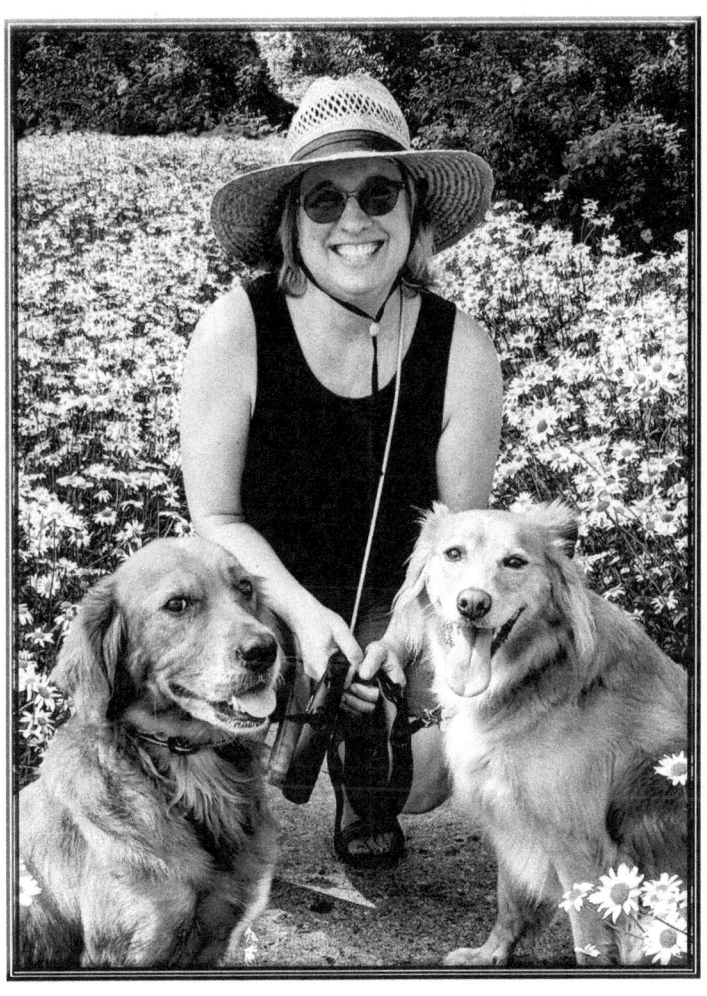

Deb strolls in a neighborhood garden with adopted dogs Heidi and Zoey.

Connect with Deb

Visit **www.debkline.com** and learn more about Deb including her energy work, music, art, community outreach, and more.

www.ingramcontent.com/pod-product-compliance
Lightning Source LLC
Chambersburg PA
CBHW072143100526
44589CB00015B/2060